The Emotional Labour of Nursing

Its impact on interpersonal relations, management
and the educational environment in nursing

Pam Smith, BNurs MSc PhD RNT

Director of Nursing Research & Development
District Nursing Adviser's Department,
Bloomsbury and Islington District Health Authority

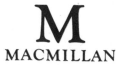

M

MACMILLAN

1

First published 1992 by
MACMILLAN EDUCATION LTD
Houndmills, Basingstoke, Hampshire RG21 2XS
and London
Companies and representatives
throughout the world

ISBN 0–333–55699–2

A catalogue record for this book is available
from the British Library.

Printed in Hong Kong

Contents

Foreword

Christine Hancock,
General Secretary, Royal College of Nursing

Pam Smith's analysis of the socialisation of student nurses is vivid, moving and challenging. She uses a wealth of personal anecdotes from student nurses as well as her own, very perceptive observations to record the changing responses of students to patients and to their work. At its most extreme, the process of socialisation reduces the fresh-eyed first-year student who identifies with the emotional needs of patients to a cynical and disillusioned practitioner preoccupied with getting through the 'real' tasks of bed baths and medication.

Pam Smitch demonstrates that nurse education has failed to value the emotional labour of nursing and to teach students how to give emotionally explicit care without burning themselves out. Because this fundamental aspect of nursing is neglected within the curriculum, students themselves fail to value it, tending to believe that 'absolute facts' are more important.

Project 2000 will relieve many of the pressures on student nurses which come from the weight of responsibility they carry for direct patient care. However, nurse educators will still need to respond to the challenge thrown down by Pam Smith's book and look hard at their teaching programmes in order to prepare and support student nurses better.

Pam Smith's work confirms that many of the distancing techniques observed by Isabel Menzies in the 1960s are still being practised today to help nurses cope with the pain of nursing. Her study pinpoints the key role of the ward sister in setting the emotional tone of the ward. The ward sister's management style determines whether the student's individuality is encouraged or repressed, whether the student can resist the weight of the nursing hierarchy and whether, therefore, they can learn to harness their own personal resources to meet the individual needs of patients.

I hope that Pam Smith's book will be widely read by ward sisters and charge nurses, by managers and by educators. It is a challenge to us all.

Preface

I clearly remember the incident that finally triggered me to make an in-depth study of nursing. I was working at the time as a nurse teacher in elderly care. I had chosen that specialty because I thought it would be free from the high-tech heroics of the acute medical and surgical wards. Nurses rather than doctors would provide care rather than cure and emphasise person rather than patienthood.

Full of enthusiasm, I redesigned the content of the teaching programme to reflect patient-centred care based on nursing rather than medical criteria. I substituted sessions on disease and treatment with those on interpersonal relationships and ways of maintaining patients' daily living activities. Some sessions were used to look at ways of prioritising care around patients' needs rather than routines.

Imagine my discomfort when a student told me that she had been reprimanded by the ward sister* for agreeing to help a patient bathe and wash her hair in the afternoon rather than the morning. The student had been so excited at being encouraged to give patients choice that the sister's displeasure at having her ward routines disrupted came as quite of a shock.

The incident provoked in me a number of questions. What was it that compelled the sister to insist that certain tasks were completed by a regular time? Was it unreasonable to put patients at the centre of care when human life expectancy limited the 'triumphs' of modern medicine? Most importantly, I felt I had let the student down. Was I teaching to strive for ideals that, although promoted by popular nursing ideologies, were inappropriate to their everyday realities? Somehow I didn't think so. But I had to find out why and how.

Eventually I was given the opportunity to seek out some of the answers to my questions by a progressive nurse manager who saw the value of an in-depth study of the subjective experiences of student nurses during training. As a participant observer I had a

---

*'Ward sister' and 'sister' are equivalent to 'charge nurse'.

unique opportunity to talk to nurses and to be allowed back in to the world of the ward. I experienced at first hand some of the contrasts and contradictions of learning to care and was led to feel it, along with the nurses, as labour of an emotional kind.

Discussions after a sociology seminar with friends brought Arlie Hochschild's study of flight attendants to my attention. I would like to thank Anne Karp who told me about that study, *The Managed Heart*, which introduced me to the notion of 'emotional labour' as part of work. I would also like to thank Arlie Hochschild, with whom I discussed the first draft of this book. Her sociological imagination facilitated me not only in the writing of the book but also to extending my understanding of the notion of emotional labour as applied to nursing.

Jane Salvage encouraged my early efforts at transforming a thesis into a manuscript and Joe Hanlon gave invaluable comments on the final drafts. To both my thanks. Also to Dave Wield, Maureen Mackintosh, Naomi Richman, Teresa Smart, Nicki Thorogood and many other friends, particularly in the thesis days, for lots of emotional labour along the way.

I would also like to thank Sally Gee, John Gee and Bridget Smith, who provided me with comfortable accommodation and conversation during long days of writing.

My colleagues have also played an important part in showing interest and support for the book. I am also appreciative of understanding managers who allowed me to take leave in order to write both thesis and book.

Finally, thanks to the student nurses, sisters, teachers and staff nurses in the study for showing me what it means to care. Since completing the research, changes within the health service, nurse education and the impact of caring for people with Acquired Immune Deficiency Syndrome (AIDS) have increased the emotional load on nurses, but not the resources. Their caring capacity is stretched to the limit. The detail, but not the spirit, of my research might have been different if I were conducting it now. But the message remains the same: caring is work and requires skill and resources.

Unfortunately, I am not able to thank the people in my study by name for reasons of confidentiality. But to you all my thanks, especially the four ward sisters and the director of nursing at 'City' Hospital. This book is dedicated to you.

Pam Smith
20 February 1991

Acknowledgements

I should like to thank the following people, who have contributed to the production of this book in a variety of ways. Firstly, I wish to thank Dr Sally Redfern who supervised the original thesis and Dr Martin Bland who advised on the statistics.

The illustrations were compiled from a number of sources. Thank you to the Department of Health, Cancer Relief Macmillan Fund and Marie Curie Cancer Care for permission to use their advertisements. Flashback, Soho, supplied the Rank Organisation still from *Carry On Matron*. The cartoons were originally drawn by Cath Jackson as part of a series for Jane Salvage's book *The Politics of Nursing* (Heinemann). Thank you to both for permission to reproduce them here. A number of individuals contributed time and expertise to produce the photographs. They include Chris Priest of Magpie Reprographics and Liz Ashton Hill who took the photographs, the senior nurses who advised on locations and sources and the subjects who agreed to be featured.

Thanks also go to The English National Board of Nursing, Midwifery and Health Visiting, for permission to reproduce extracts from the General Nursing Council's 1977 training syllabus and student nurse assessment form. I would also like to thank Dr Joan Fretwell for permission to use and reproduce her Ward Learning Environment Rating Questionnaire.

I am grateful to Sheila Fawell for permission to include an extract from her study of student nurses undertaking their psychiatric experience.

Finally, I should like to thank Rex Parry, Isobel Munday and Ian Kingston of Macmillan Education for their patience and thoroughness in preparing the book for publication.

Every effort has been made to trace all the copyright holders, but if any have been inadvertently overlooked the publishers will be pleased to make the necessary arrangements at the first opportunity.

1 Introduction

'The little things'

While making beds with a student nurse soon after she was allocated to an elderly care hospital, I remember her being close to tears because she felt that the old people were being treated like sacks of potatoes – hauled in and out of bed at the beginning and end of their day with no control over their destiny. Other students talked more positively about their experiences of elderly care, discovering that it was 'the little things' that made the qualitative difference to patients' lives; little things such as dressing in their own clothes, manicuring their nails, making sure their hearing aids worked and their glasses were clean. As one student put it, in the elderly ward, the functioning hearing aid was just as much a lifeline to survival as the intravenous infusion to the postoperative patient on the acute surgical ward. On the elderly ward, the high-tech heroics were set aside and 'the little things' became all important.

From my own experiences as a young patient and student nurse I recalled that in acute wards, too, it was 'the little things' that made the qualitative difference, especially as to how I felt. The nursing assistant who, when I was a patient, broke hospital rules to bring me an Easter egg. The sister in the outpatient department who noticed me shivering in a wheelchair and tucked me up in a blanket. My own nurse teacher who visited students on the wards and encouraged us to talk about our patients as individuals rather than cases. I reflected that all of these people had shown personal interest in me and made me feel safe and cared for in an environment that was otherwise threatening, rigid and hierarchical.

But these 'little things' or 'gestures of caring' are difficult to capture and slip by unnoticed in the daily routines and hustle and bustle of ward life, except when the patient is there for life. Then the absence of these 'little things' is stark evidence of the

1

lack of care[1]. So why then when they make such a difference to how people feel do we refer to these things as 'little'? One explanation lies in the stereotyping of care as women's 'natural' work which keeps it invisible and undervalued and on the margins of high-tech medically defined work[2].

The reproduction of gender stereotypes is no better demonstrated than in the public images and perceptions of nurses and nursing. Attitude surveys reveal, for example, that the public identify 'alertness to the needs of others' as the mark of both the good woman and the good nurse (Oakley, 1984). These attitudes reflect the patriarchal nature of nursing's origins, enshrined in the powerful image of Florence Nightingale on the back of the British £10 note, tending to sick and dying soldiers[3].

Nurse recruitment posters convey the predominant image of nurses, usually women, as carers rather than technicians; special people who make a difference. 'Patients remember nurses' one poster states; or another showing a little girl in a nurse's uniform holding her bandaged teddy bear: 'the best nurses have the essential qualifications before they go to school'. In other words, caring is portrayed as intuitive, instinctive, as something you're born with by virtue of your gender. Yet another poster advertising the nursing services of a cancer charity shows a child's drawing of a smiling nurse. The caption reads: 'Mummy said she had cancer. Daddy got very upset. The nurse made them both feel better'.

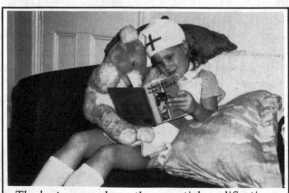

*The best nurses have the essential qualifications
before they go to School*

*This illustration is based on a DHSS recruitment
advert from the early 1980s*
(Source: Pam Smith)

2

"MUMMY SAID SHE HAD CANCER.

DADDY GOT VERY UPSET.

THE NURSE MADE THEM BOTH FEEL BETTER."

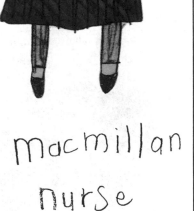

A Macmillan Nurse helps care for people with cancer. We need your support to help her do even more. Send your donations to 15/19 Britten St, London SW3 3TZ.

Cancer Relief
Macmillan Fund
Living with cancer

Recent recruitment campaigns show that these images prevail. Young women are still most likely to appear in the recruitment posters and although a variety of technical images are presented (such as nursing a patient in head traction or tapping into a computer), the central message is that nursing is about people and ensuring the welfare of patients and their families.

An advertisement for the Marie Curie cancer charity shows three powerful images of a nurse comforting the distressed wife of a cancer patient. She is performing the 'little things': holding, talking and preparing a cup of tea. The nurse seemingly performs these tasks effortlessly, with little demand on herself and for little material reward. Part of the wording reads: 'People sometimes ask me how I can do this, nursing people who are terminally ill. But you have only to take the hand of someone who's caring for a dying relative. Someone who's really desperate to rest. You can almost feel the relief easing its way through them. Then you know it's worthwhile'.

What is care?

But what is care? How can it be defined to go beyond these powerful images of nurses as caring (smiling, holding, talking) women, making things better for others? A number of feminist

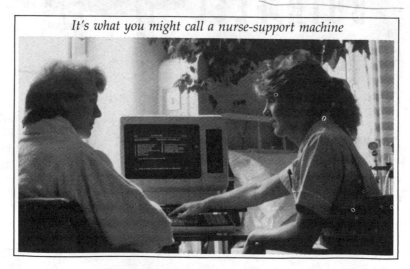

It's what you might call a nurse-support machine

(Source: Department of Health)

4

66It wasn't the cancer

patient who needed me it was the relatives.

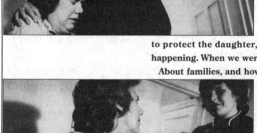

When I arrived at the house the patient was asleep upstairs. I was immediately concerned about his wife. She looked as if she hadn't seen her bed for a week, which she probably hadn't. Her daughter was just leaving as I arrived.

They were obviously very close, but I got the impression that the mother was still trying to protect the daughter, to shield her from what was happening. When we were alone, we talked. Just talked. About families, and how quickly things change. Sometimes a cup of tea is the best medicine in the world.

People sometimes ask me how I can do this, nursing people who are terminally ill. But you only have to take the hand of someone who's caring for a dying relative. Someone who's really desperate to rest. You can almost feel the relief easing its way through them. Then you know that it's worthwhile.

Every night Marie Curie nurses stay in the homes of people with cancer. They bring relief to the patients. And comfort and support to the relatives and friends who are caring for them. Please help us to continue this work.

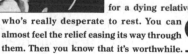
5

sociologists have attempted to answer this question (Stacey, 1981; Graham, 1983; Ungerson, 1983a, 1983b, 1990). Graham, for example, describes caring as both labour and love, caring for and caring about, doing and feeling. She says: 'everyday conversations about caring are . . . conversations about feelings. When we talk about caring for someone we are talking about our emotions' (Graham, 1983 p.15).

In general, caring relationships are those involving and defining women in both the public and private domain. Throughout the life-cycle women care for children, partners, relatives who are sick, handicapped or elderly[4]. They reproduce these caring activities in the public arena of work[5]. But differences occur in the affective domain where feelings of love, concern and empathy are in danger of being replaced by 'social distance' (Graham, 1983).

Nicky James (1989), a nurse sociologist who spent five months as a participant observer in a hospice, chooses to describe care as labour. She found that the demands of emotion work with the dying and their families could be equally as hard as physical and technical labour, but not so readily recognised and valued. James concludes: 'the management of emotions has many of the connotations associated with labour as productive work but also the sense of labour as difficult, requiring effort and sometimes pain. It demands that the labourer gives something of themselves and not just a formulaic response'.

She describes how emotions such as grief, anger, loss, despair and frustration were painful to watch and awkward to respond to, particularly as they did not fit in with standard ideas of workplace skills. But they were anticipated and seen as appropriate responses in coming to terms with death. Sometimes however, nurses would choose to concentrate on the physical aspects of the patient's care in order to avoid difficult relationships. When this happened, the 'love' part of the work was lost (James, 1986).

Arlie Hochschild (1983), an American sociologist, also makes conceptual links between care, feelings and emotions. In her study of flight attendants, Hochschild uses the term 'labour' rather than care to describe the emotional component of their work (smiling, friendly, kind, courteous) which is required as part of their job and has explicit monetary value both for themselves and the airline.

6

Hochschild defines emotional labour as: the induction or suppression of feeling in order to sustain an outward appearance that produces in others a sense of being cared for in a convivial safe place (p.7). She goes on to say that jobs which involve emotional labour share three characteristics:

1. Face to face or voice contact with the public.
2. They require the worker to produce an emotional state in another, e.g. gratitude, fear.
3. They allow the employer through training and supervision to exercise a degree of control over the emotional activities of the employees (p. 147).

Thus, according to Hochschild, emotional labour is the occupational equivalent of emotion work/management which is done in a private context. It is sold for a wage and has exchange value. Because jobs with high components of emotional labour are most likely to be female occupations, gender stereotypes and expectations are reproduced in the workplace. Whether emotional labour is undertaken in the workplace or as emotion work/management in the home, it is guided by what Hochschild calls 'feeling rules'. Feeling rules are the scripts or moral stances that guide our action. They come from within us, the reaction of others and social conventions.

Emotion work/management/labour intervenes to shape our actions when there is a gap between what we actually feel and what we think we should feel. Take the feeling of 'anger' for example. 'Perhaps women are not any less aggressive than men' Flax, a feminist writer suggests, 'we may just express our aggression in different, culturally sanctioned (and partially disguised or denied) ways' (Flax, 1987). In order to express our feelings in 'culturally sanctioned ways' Hochschild suggests that there are two kinds of emotion work: surface and deep acting.

In surface acting we consciously change our outer expression in order to make our inner feelings correspond to how we appear. Deep acting requires us to change our feelings from the inside using a variety of methods such as imaging, verbal and physical prompting so that the feelings we want to feel show on our face. Both feeling rules and emotion work may be unconscious or semi-conscious.

7

The emotional labour of care

But is emotional labour as a concept the same as care? What are the similarities and differences and the inherent contradictions of treating emotional labour as a commodity ?

I apply the concept of emotional labour to nursing because nurses are expected to be emotionally caring and display emotional styles similar to those of flight attendants.

I first experienced caring as labour during interviews with students and patients when the language that they used and the feelings that they expressed conveyed a sense of the sheer emotional work required to sustain the traditional image of smiling nurses, holding patients' hands. During one such interview a student described the following incident. 'I've had times when I've been with another nurse and we've been changing a patient's bed and he's shouted at her or been rude or something. Well the procedure goes on as if nothing has happened. And when we've finished she just drifts off. And I actually go after her and say "Are you alright? I would have been very unhappy if he'd said that to me". I think it's so important that we notice each other's distress so that we don't have to cry alone in a corner'.

As this account demonstrates, nurses not only laboured emotionally for patients, but also for each other. The ward sister was the key person who set the tone for the caring climate on her ward. As one student explained 'if sister cares then I don't need to take the whole caring attitude of the whole ward on my shoulders'.

Nursing and care

It is interesting to examine the way nursing leaders and educationalists conceptualise care. A look at the literature shows an increasing emphasis on the emotional aspects of caring and its promotion as distinctly nursing work since the influential Briggs report (DHSS, 1972).

Jean (now Baroness) McFarlane, a prominent nurse academic, in a keynote address to the Royal College of Nursing, maintained that the words 'nursing' and 'caring' have similar roots. She says: 'Caring signifies a feeling of concern, of interest, of oversight, with a view to protection. Nursing means . . . to nourish and cherish (McFarlane, 1976, p. 189).

McFarlane wanted to see an end to the nurse as the doctor's handmaiden and the emergence of a new role in which caring was pre-eminent. By describing nursing in terms of 'helping, assisting, serving, caring for' patients, McFarlane was seeking to raise the status of so-called basic tasks to the level of unique nursing skills. In a subsequent paper, she provided a philosophy and work method called the nursing process, to do this (McFarlane, 1977). The nursing process, regarded by many as an American import, promotes a people- rather than task-orientated approach to patients and raises the profile of emotional care at the same time that, as Hochschild notes, the growth of the service sector and 'people jobs' has made communication and encounter the central work relationship[6].

Changes in the structure and knowledge base of nurse education proposed by the United Kingdom Central Council's Project 2000 (UKKC, 1986) and innovations such as primary nursing described by Jane Salvage (1990) as part of the 'new nursing', build on the nursing process philosophy and work method to emphasise people-centred care rather than patients and disease[7].

What the nursing leadership has failed to do, however, is to grapple with the conceptual complexity of defining care, especially in relation to its emotional components and demands. An important implication of raising the profile of emotional care can be seen in the light of research undertaken in a London hospital over thirty years ago by Isabel Menzies, a British psychoanalyst. Brought in to investigate some of the reasons why students were leaving nursing, she believed that high anxiety levels were partly responsible. Menzies saw the task-orientated way in which nursing care was organised as a defence against that anxiety (Menzies, 1960). She wrote:

> The nursing service attempts to protect the nurse from the anxiety of her relation with the patient by splitting up her contacts with them. The total workload of a ward or department is broken down into lists of tasks, each of which is allocated to a particular nurse.

In the light of Menzies' findings, the nursing process, with its explicit commitment to the development of nurse–patient relationships, puts the nurse at risk of increasing her anxiety by removing the protection provided by task-orientated care.

The nursing leadership also failed to address why many nurses favoured high-tech, medically defined nursing. MacFarlane, for example, believed that an early job analysis of hospital nursing by Goddard (1953) in which the physical, technical and affective aspects of nursing had been distinguished, emphasised the status of technical over physical and affective nursing. Fretwell (1982) more realistically points out that the distinction reflected the existing medical division of labour and hierarchy within nursing. MacFarlane's reaction was typical of the curious lack of feminist perspectives brought to bear on the position of nurses by its leaders. Issues such as the stereotyping of care as women's 'natural work' (encapsulated by the recruitment posters) and the gender division of labour within the health service and the patriarchal power relations between doctors (predominantly men) and nurses (predominantly women) were not addressed in these official versions of nursing[8]. *The politics of nursing*, written by Jane Salvage (1985), is an important departure from the traditional nursing texts in which she addresses some of these fundamental issues[9].

The body–mind dichotomy

Concepts of care are fraught with contrasts and contradictions. Is it labour or is it love? Is it natural or is it a skill? Is it about feelings or tasks? Does it come from the heart, the head or the hand? Is it guided by mind or body? Or should caring be seen as an integrated whole ?

Hochschild's work is sometimes criticised because it is seen as perpetuating the body–mind dichotomy, which has its origins in positivism, western dualism and what Mary O'Brien calls 'malestream' thought[10]. Pat Benner, an American Professor of Nursing, applies a philosophical approach to the concept of care, which she says transcends the body–mind split and enables connection and concern between nurse and patient. Emotions are seen as the key to this connection because 'they allow the person to be engaged or involved in the situation .... The alienated, detached view of emotions, as unruly bodily responses that must be controlled actually cuts the person off from being involved in the situation in a complete way' (Benner and Wrubel, 1989).

Views such as these represent a trend over the past decade amongst nurses in the USA and Europe to move to a more holistic approach to care and away from 'a nation's blind embrace of high tech medicine' (Gordon, 1988).

The politics of care

As concerns for cost-effectiveness and efficiency sweep the British health service and budgets are finely tuned to respond to the purchaser–provider divide, the 'little things' are in double danger. On the one hand, nurses working under increasing pressure will find even less time to do 'the little things' for patients. On the other, the increase in monitoring and standard setting may focus more on quantitative measures rather than qualities of care. At what price is care, since emotional care is not easily costed?

Hochschild found in her study that certain conditions, such as reduction in staffing levels and quicker turn-round of flights militated against the production of emotional labour. Similarly, in the NHS the cut-back on resources circumscribes the amount of emotional labour that nurses are able to do. Nurses' salaries unlike those of flight attendants, do not explicitly reflect payment for the emotional component of their labour.

A recent recruitment poster gave a mixed message. On the one hand it reassured prospective nurses that although they were unlikely to be attracted to the job for the money, they would be well paid for their skills. On the other hand, it emphasised that they could expect emotional rewards *as well as* financial ones. In other words, the emotional rewards came as an added bonus for working in one of the most 'emotionally satisfying professions' (see illustration on p. 12).

It is interesting to speculate as to whether the privatisation of the NHS will lead to a commercialisation of nurses' emotional labour in the private health industry. Already the images used for advertising private health insurance bear similiarities to those used by the airline industry for attracting custom. Like the recruitment posters and charity advertisements, the nurse is portrayed as the key carer, smiling and helpful to the patient and their family (see illustration on p. 13).

11

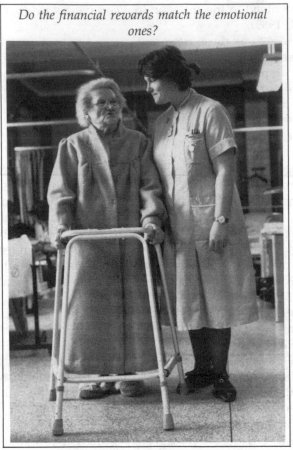

Do the financial rewards match the emotional ones?

This illustration is based on a DoH recruitment advertisement
(Source: Liz Ashton Hill)

But a contradictory trend is emerging in the rapidly changing health service which marginalises care even further from medically defined work. A recent *Guardian* article, which describes an elderly ward staffed by untrained carers, is an example of this (Brindle, 1990). Nurse training is criticised for being too formal and nurses too wedded to routine to provide the 'caring touch' for elderly long-stay residents. The technical needs of the residents are provided by a visiting nurse who is described as doing the 'tricky dressings' and complicated medicines. The untrained carers on the other hand describe themselves as 'just

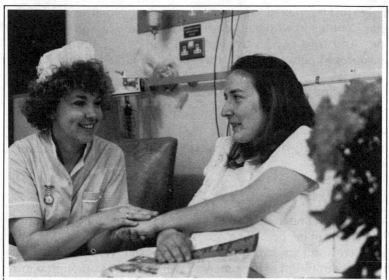

Feel confident that when you or a member of your family need hospital treatment, you'll enjoy comfort, privacy and individual attention.

This illustration is based on a private health insurance advert
(Source: Liz Ashton Hill)

in the new cost-effective health service which drives a sharp division between caring, 'making people happy', and their technical requirements, marginalising 'the little things' the caring gestures, from the technical skills.

Emotional labour costs

As this account from an interview with a student nurse illustrates, patients and their families value and need caring nurses, but these skills that Benner calls connection and involvement require teaching and learning, both to protect the nurse and heal the patient.

I asked the student to describe any incidents that she had found particularly stressful during her training. She told me about her time on the paediatric ward when she became involved with a young child and her family.

13

There just happened to be a patient on the paediatric ward at the time, a little girl who had cancer and for some reason she took to me. And in a good way and in a bad way I think this was encouraged because she loathed being in hospital. She was six.

Q. How good and bad?

She had a lot of chemotherapy and she died in the end, but it was good I think because she took to me, her mother did and her family did. But bad because it all became a bit too much really.

Q. In what way too much?

Well stressful really. I didn't say at work but I should have done. It was silly of me because there is a very highly esteemed teacher up there and I am sure she would have been very helpful now I think about it. But at the time you want to look as though you're coping. I mean the trained staff are there but they all knew that this child had taken to me so much and I was obviously being very useful to her making hospital not quite perhaps so unbearable as it had been, but it was quite a strain. I think it was from her mother more than her. Obviously her mother was very anxious.

I'm surprised nobody actually said to me 'are you managing, is it alright?' I think they forget about that side of nursing. They think 'Oh yeah, you're a nurse, you can manage'. But you can't really. I mean we're still pretty young. Outwardly you might be managing, but you know I used to go home and cry my eyes out sometimes. It was dreadful. But I've found that at work well you've almost got to be, well people expect you to be happy and not cross. And you can't be cross even though you feel like wringing someone's neck! You've got to be reasonably under control and of course everybody suffers when you go home.

I think you learn to stop that, you learn to switch off and be different, forget about work when you go home, I mean you've got to.

Q. And do you think you learn that?

I think you do, but through trial and error.

First, the student recognises the importance of giving emotional support to a child and her family and the need for

14

'connection and involvement'. But she also describes how she was pulled down by her lack of skill in handling her involvement in the absence of trained staff who recognised and supported the emotional cost of caring. She recognises that, as a nurse, she is expected to be happy rather than cross and to manage and cope with extremes of feelings. As these expectations come from her seniors, she consequently expects them of herself. Like Hochschild's flight attendants, she must induce or suppress her own feelings, some would say subordinate them, to make others feel cared for and safe, irrespective of how she feels herself. She learns through 'trial and error' to 'switch off' and 'forget about work' when she goes home. But is this through surface acting to the point that she can no longer remain involved with patients other than at a superficial level, at risk of becoming detached and alienated? Or can she learn through experience and systematic training to recognise and use her feelings to remain therapeutically involved both for herself and the patient?

Hochschild's findings suggest that she can. One group of flight attendants that she studied received intensive training in the use of deep and surface acting to manage their emotions in given situations. Older more experienced workers were found to be particularly adept at deep acting which allowed them to distinguish between their 'personal' and 'work' selves, develop a 'healthy' estrangement between self and work role and prevent burn out.

The acting techniques employed by the flight attendants seem feasible for the duration of a flight, but nurses have to sustain emotional involvement for much longer periods. Often they develop their own emotional labour strategies[11], some of which are positive but many of which evolve to protect them from a range of feelings: guilt, fear, failure and anger, to name but a few.

How do Hochschild's notions of deep and surface acting apply to nurses' accounts of their presentation of self to the outside world?

Hochschild's suggestion that we manage our emotions according to feeling rules represented, for me, a framework for interpreting the empirical reality I encountered through the students' accounts and my own field observations. The students quoted above clearly appeared to be managing their feelings, whether it was to carry on as if nothing had happened when a patient had shouted or been rude to them, or to make a little girl's stay in hospital not seem quite so unbearable, despite feeling personally upset by her condition.

The patients in these accounts were the recipients of the students' emotional labour. But what did other patients expect of nurses? How did their expectations contribute to the feeling rules that shaped their relationships with nurses?

Everybody's ideal

When I asked patients to describe a 'good' nurse they were more likely to talk about attitudes and feelings rather than technical competence.

Forty-four different words or phrases were used by the patients to describe 'ideal' and 'real' nurses. Only six of these words or phrases referred to functional rather than affective attributes. Coser (1962) who designed the original interview agenda (see Methodological Appendix, p. 160) reported similar findings. Words used to describe nurses' functional attributes included: efficient, observant, alert and 'capable of doing their job'. One patient combined both functional and affective attributes by expecting nurses to be 'caring but efficient'. As we shall see in Chapter 5, ward sisters also distinguished between nurses' functional and affective attributes. The caring (i.e. emotional) aspects of nursing were clearly seen as distinct but complementary to and underpinning the functional (i.e. efficient, observant, capable, alert) aspects.

Kindness, helpfulness and patience were the affective or caring aspects most frequently used to describe the City Hospital nurses. Nurses were said to keep patients happy by being cheerful, loving, considerate, friendly and understanding and made them feel at home. Talking, listening, showing interest and sympathy all featured as examples of the ideal nurse. As one patient concluded:

A nurse has to be aware of the patient's condition and how to tackle it. She has to have a nursing manner which requires a lot of patience and forethought and to try and relieve pain and suffering not by medical means but by compassion.

16

This quotation is interesting because the patient has a clear view that a nursing manner requires patience, forethought and compassion to relieve pain and suffering, which are distinct from medical means.

The nurse as emotional labourer

From these and other data it emerges that patients, like the students, realise that nurses have to work emotionally on themselves in order to care for patients. This view of care as emotional labour suggests that, potentially, patients are recognising that caring is more than just part of the package of women's work.

The following quotations offer some interesting perspectives on the nurse as emotional labourer.

The first patient, a young man in his thirties, was a trained laboratory technician. He had had a lot of hospital experience, both as a worker and patient, and had even been a student nurse for a brief period. His background and interests therefore gave him some interesting insights. He said:

As a nurse you are more at the beck and call of the public than in a supermarket. I tell the nurse don't forget you're only human. You see them when the patient keeps ringing the bell and they grimace to themselves. Then they go up to the patient all smiles.

Here he compares the nurse with another service sector worker, the supermarket assistant. The difference between the two, he believes, is that the nurse is more vulnerable to the demands of the public. He closely observes the reaction of the nurse to the 'demanding' patient who keeps on ringing his call bell for assistance. She grimaces, irritated that yet again she is being called. But she can't show the patient she is irritated so she transforms her grimace into smiles as she approaches him. The patient who is recounting this story clearly recognises that this transformation costs 'superhuman' effort by reminding the nurses that they are only human.

The second patient is also in his thirties and has had multiple hospital admissions for a chronic condition. As I speak to him he implies he has been hurt by getting too close to nurses in the

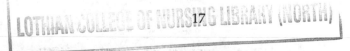

past. He values those nurses who make him feel at home but he is also aware that 'care can be dangerous if you are emotional about patients, you can't let it affect you, it's got to be platonic'. The view that being emotional is dangerous and that platonic care is preferable is interesting in the light of an analysis of emotional labour. The importance of making the patient feel that care is safe rather than dangerous again shows that managing emotions requires skill over and above 'natural' caring qualities, and is different to love.

Patients, like students, identified caring as the emotional side of nursing as being distinct but complementary to and underpinning the functional (efficient, observant, capable, alert) attributes of the 'ideal' nurse. Some patients recognised that nurses had to work emotionally on themselves (undertake emotional labour) in order to appear caring at all times. This observation is of immense importance, because it potentially recognises that caring is more than just part of the package of women's work and requires specialist learning to produce in others a sense of feeling cared for in a safe place.

In more recent research, Hochschild (1989) focused on emotional life at home and the different strategies adopted by working parents for dividing domestic labour and gratitude in the home. She shows how gender ideologies may either reinforce or conflict with reality. Feeling rules come into play which guide emotion work to produce a gender-specific strategy to cope with the conflict. Hochschild concludes that one of the most important costs to women is that society devalues the work of the home and sees women as inferior because they do devalued work.

What then are the implications of these findings for nurses, given that nursing reproduces many of the traditional female roles and domestic tasks in the workplace? What is the fit between gender and occupational ideologies? Do conflicts arise and if so what feelings are generated? Do feeling rules come into play to guide emotion work and produce strategies to cope with these conflicts? If so, how do they manifest themselves?

In the seven chapters that follow, I draw on extensive case study material to examine some of these questions in relation to nurses as emotional labourers. The material is used to construct a series of close-up portraits, nurses' own accounts and reflections on the nature of nursing and caring. As we progress through each chapter, looking at the viability of emotional labour

18

as a concept, nurses' different emotional styles, the students' training trajectories and how they learn to care, the role of the ward sister in setting the emotional tone, the legitimisation of emotional labour and the forms it takes between both nurses and nurses on the one hand and nurses and patients on the other we shall also see the strategies nurses adopt both to keep in touch and to protect themselves from their feelings.

Perspectives are also offered on the content and structure of nurse training, which are of particular relevance to planning and implementing Project 2000.

In summary then, this is a book about nurses and nursing which goes beyond the popular and professional rhetoric to examine the notion of emotional labour as a component of caring, how nurses care and learn to care and its effects on carers and the cared for.

2 Putting their toe in the water: selecting, testing and expecting nurses to care

Research subjects, settings and methods

I began my study as the demographic time bomb and the nursing recruitment crisis began to challenge the assumption that there would always be an unlimited supply of young women motivated to become nurses[1].

The setting for the research was a typical British teaching hospital where, as one study showed, most of the direct nursing (about 75 per cent) was provided by nurses in training (Moores and Moult, 1979). These nurses were usually between 18 and 21 years old and faced a range of life and death issues in the prime of their lives[2].

In order to gather my data and gain insights into the research setting I worked as a nurse in a number of wards and attended classes in the school of nursing. In this way I was able to re-experience the world of the student nurse and to construct their three-year training trajectories (see Appendix A). I also conducted in-depth interviews with nurses and patients.

In addition I distributed over 500 student questionnaires on the ward learning environment. The questionnaire, developed and tested by Joan Fretwell (1985) was based on her own research in nurse training schools and gave me very useful complementary information. It enabled me to cover a much wider population of students and wards beyond the subjects of my in-depth study (see Methodological Appendix).

Who train as nurses?

The nursing work force at 'City' Hospital[3] was typical of most teaching hospitals as described above. By far the largest group were the trainee nurses, aged between 18 and 21, on the front-line of patient care. They also best fitted the public's image of the nurse as 'young lady' or 'good woman' and Nightingale's descendant who was vocationally motivated, obedient and subservient to both medical and nursing superiors.

To what extent this image of the nurse was ever an accurate or representative perception is open to speculation since historically the nursing workforce in Britain is not a homogeneous group (Bellaby and Oribabor, 1980). Their class, gender and racial composition may vary according to grade, specialty, institution or region in which they work. But the predominant image of the nurse as white, middle-class and female prevails and affects the content of their work, training, and public and professional expectations and prospects[4].

How then did nurse managers and educators in charge of recruitment at City Hospital maintain the student workforce in the image of Nightingale i.e. white, middle-class and female?

The job prospectus

One way of maintaining the image was through the job prospectus. The first page read:

It is the aim of the hospital to create a friendly and happy atmosphere in which nurses can more easily care for the physical and psychological needs of the patient and fulfil their desire to be of service to others.

Of interest here is the commitment to the creation of a friendly and happy atmosphere, but also that such an atmosphere facilitates caring. Caring is clearly identified as what nurses do, but more importantly it is underpinned by the assumption that caring *fulfils* a nurse's *desire* to be of *service* to others (my emphasis). Like Hochschild's applicants to become flight attendants, prospective nurses were being introduced to the 'rules of the game' through the language of the prospectus, even before interview.

The 'rules' were compounded by photographs contained in the prospectus which showed images of young white women engaged in a number of professional and personal activities: talking with patients and colleagues, studying in the library, playing tennis and dressmaking. Images of male and black nurses were noticeably absent. More recent versions of the

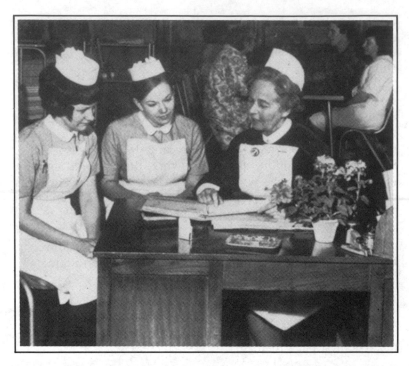

Recruitment images at the beginning of the research portrayed student nurses and ward sisters as white and female.

prospectus, like the national recruitment campaigns, include such images. Recreational activities are more varied, and tennis and dressmaking have given way to cultural and culinary pursuits about town. The new prospectus, however, still retains much of the language of the earlier version promoting nursing as care and concern.

Selection procedures

City Hospital was popular amongst prospective student nurses, and six times the number of candidates required to fill the 180 places applied annually. Thus the nurse recruiters found themselves with a large pool of applicants from which they could select students judged to possess the necessary qualities, not only to become nurses, but more specifically to train at City.

These qualities included working with people and academic ability, as measured by obtaining Ordinary Level passes in the

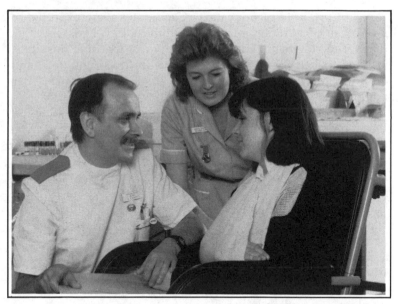

In recent recruitment images, male and black nurses are no longer absent: staff nurse with student and patient.
(Source: Chris Priest)

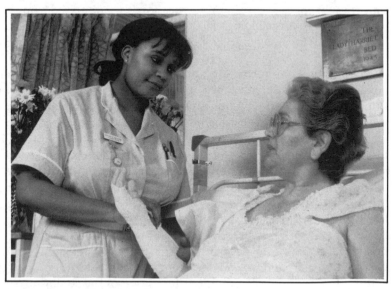

Student nurse with patient.
(Source: Chris Priest)

General Certificate of Education. Candidates were expected to have obtained a minimum of five Ordinary Level passes.

Nurse recruiters at City, in line with most teaching hospitals, not only looked for 'personal' qualities in their candidates but for a higher educational standard than the national entry requirements of two Ordinary Level passes[5].

During interviews I began to note how the two types of selection criteria presented students with seemingly contradictory versions of nursing. On the one hand they were selected because of their interest in and experience of working with people. On the other, they were expected to have reached a good educational standard with priority being given to those students who had obtained passes in biological subjects. An analysis of the students' entry qualifications showed that the majority of them had obtained an Ordinary Level pass in biology and almost a third of them had also obtained an Advanced Level pass in the subject. The number of people with passes in socially orientated subjects, such as history and sociology, was much lower.

The differences in defining the two types of selection criteria implied that a student's interest and experience in working with people came as part of the personal and experiential package that they brought with them as vocationally orientated young women, whereas the biological knowledge required to nurse had to be learnt formally and validated both before and during training.

The emphasis on recruiting applicants who had already been engaged in paid or voluntary 'people' work ensured, in one tutor's words, that the prospective students had 'put their toe in the water' as a sort of test to prove to them that 'not everyone was nice'. If they had passed their test and still wanted to nurse, then in the tutor's eyes there was a good chance that these students would maintain outward composure in their future encounters with patients who were not being 'nice'. That nursing as people work was treated as a central issue during interview was expressed by one student who said, 'when you come for your interview, they ask if you're interested in people, do you like talking to people, do they matter?' Her own view was that 'if people don't matter, then you can't do nursing'.

But when it came to academic criteria, one of the senior nurse recruiters told me that the reason why students at City were required to have more education certificates for entry into nursing compared with national standards was because of the 'academically demanding' environment where they would be working. I also read a statement in an educational report that said the City recruiters wanted 'articulate' student nurses who would understand clinical medicine and be acceptable to the medical staff of a teaching hospital.

The recruiter confirmed this statement by saying candidates were chosen who would be able to work 'among professional staff' on the wards. They would have to be able to stand up in an environment that, although 'friendly', was also described as 'very hierarchical and academically demanding'. It appeared that for her this meant that 'academic' criteria went little further than secondary school biology as a basis for understanding clinical medicine so that nurses were acceptable to the medical staff. This view has resonances with the analysis that nurses' knowledge and skills revolve around the diagnostic and treatment model of care[6].

The recruiter also reasoned that, with such high expectations for City students, not all applicants were suitable for selection. The typical recruit was likely to be white, female and middle-class because of her ability to fulfil both general and specific entry criteria[7].

My own experience of coming to the City Hospital as an 'outsider' was that nurses were always friendly and put me at my ease. The hospital had a reputation for friendliness which many of the students said was the reason they had decided to nurse at the City Hospital. In this respect, the first aim of the hospital as stated in the job prospectus to create a 'friendly atmosphere' appeared to be being met.

A former patient who was now a City nurse remarked on the class characteristics of her colleagues. She said, 'I was a patient before I began training and I thought then all the girls seemed the same, very much a type and fairly upper class'.

A patient who was a public relations officer and interested in recruitment issues told me that compared to other hospitals she'd been in there was something 'special' about the City Hospital. She continued:

In my independent view it's because of the selection. The nurses are all on an even keel. They've always a smile, always got time for you and make you feel as if you're a person and not just passing through.

This patient's comment was interesting because she was essentially describing the behavioural characteristics of the City nurse as emotional labourer (on an even keel, always a smile, always got time for you) which made her feel cared for (being made to feel like a person; not just passing through). Her reference to selection confirmed the recruiter's view that selecting nurses who had already put their toe in the water with the general public ensured that they were more likely to maintain outward composure, even with patients who were not being nice.

Standing up in the City Hospital environment

The above accounts illustrate that nurses, patients and recruiters identify nursing as 'people' work in which, as Hochschild suggests, communication and encounter are central. I also began to understand that students' emotional activities were controlled by the regular practical assessments conducted during their ward placements. These assessments, like Hochschild's third characteristic of jobs which involve large components of emotional labour, provided a mechanism which allowed the employer, in this case the students' senior nurses and teachers, to exercise a degree of control over their emotional activities by regularly assessing them on their personal and professional qualities.

Although I am describing assessment procedures in operation at City, all schools of nursing were required by the training inspectorate[8] to operate similar systems. We can assume, therefore, that an analysis of systems at other schools would yield similar general findings.

The methods by which the students were tested at City were described in their plan of training as a 'series of structured and informal assessments based on detailed objectives' and 'a means by which encouragement is given to learners to *reach and maintain a high standard of nursing care throughout training*'(my emphasis). In other words, students were constantly under pressure to perform well.

The content of the assessments reflected the qualities for which the students had been selected, namely their ability to stand up in an environment that was friendly, hierarchical and academically demanding.

The detailed learning objectives for the general ward placements were concerned with acquiring competence in techniques
and procedures associated with the care of patients suffering
from specific diseases. Thus the assessment of the student's
clinical learning was based on the view of their recruiters: that
an academically demanding environment required them to
understand clinical medicine. Out of 35 general ward learning
objectives, only two dealt with patients' psychosocial needs. On
nine out of fifteen wards, students were formally assessed
usually by the trained ward staff on a number of specific
procedures such as aseptic technique and drug administration.
Students were also assessed on nursing skills related to patient
care and managing colleagues. By the time they had reached
their third year, for example, they were expected to plan,
organise and ensure quality of care given both by themselves
and their colleagues.

Other criteria on which the nurses were assessed related more
specifically to the personal qualities for which they had been
selected. They included 'personal appearance', communication
with patients and an awareness of cultural, spiritual, physical
and psychological needs. Students were also expected to be able
to prioritise care, ensure safety at all times, report and record
care given, evaluate it in terms of its effects on patients, use
teaching opportunities and evaluate their own performance.

These personal criteria on which the students were judged
were reinforced by the format of their ward reports given to
them at the end of every ward placement (see Appendix B).
Again they included appearance, punctuality, observation, forethought and management of priorities, all of which were identi-
fiable as women's 'socially expected attributes'[9].

Thus the methods by which the students were assessed
throughout training reinforced the selection criteria on which
they had been recruited, set the emotional tone of their work
and served to maintain the image of the City nurse.

As one student saw it, 'In this hospital there is a very definite
attempt to make you change your character, well, mould you
into a "City" type'. I asked her what she meant by a City 'type'.
She then described one of the ward sisters:

> She's everybody's ideal, really. She's so sophisticated, she
> always looks so calm, attractive and manages to get all the
> work done. She's very kind and considerate and yet she looks
> almost like a model.

27

Here was a description of the 'ideal' City nurse who was also the ideal emotional labourer. She maintained calm, was kind and considerate, but also competent in that she managed to get all the work done in time. Her physical appearance was important. Not only was she described as 'attractive' but almost like a 'model'.

Although the student admired this ward sister she also found the idea of emulating her daunting. This was interesting, given that to me the student physically fitted the City nurse image. She too was attractive, tall, fair and articulate. But nevertheless, she thought that 'the standards and ideals here are very high, what they want you to be. They want a lot of confidence from you, very quickly'. She then went on to refer to the ward report which she saw as 'always pushing you to be more confident'.

I then asked the student who she was referring to as 'they'. She replied:

School and the staff nurses I suppose. I don't know who formulates the ward reports, a list of all the qualities you should have. You get marks on them. It's whoever draws up that who is moulding you.

It seemed that by referring to the school and the staff nurses, i.e. those in authority, as the people who were 'moulding' the students through the ward reports, this student was identifying one aspect of the hierarchically demanding environment.

Another student described the role played by the teachers in their assessments which reinforced the hierarchical nature of their relationships. She said, 'You've got to respect a position of authority, but you shouldn't be scared like thinking "Oh god! she's going to be writing something about me". I don't want to be feeling like that about the school for three years'.

One of the tutors accurately captured the student's feelings when she said, 'they see us as their judge and jury'.

Another student experienced the ward reports as a way in which those in authority imposed a 'picture' or image of how they saw her. Like her colleague she also referred to these authority figures as 'they'. For her, 'the ward reports give you a picture of what they think you were like; not like I think I am'. She too said that confidence was the key quality on which the students were judged. 'It all depends on how confident you are. That's all they're interested in – "confidence"'.

28

But the first student added a rider which suggested that there was a fine balance between appearing confident and 'cocky' and that she found the staff's expectations difficult to interpret. 'I think it's quite difficult to see how they want you to behave as they don't want you to be "cocky" '. What she seemed to be describing here was the difference between the confidence expected of a 'young lady' able to stand up in a hierarchically demanding environment and the 'cocky' nurse able to stand up *for herself*. A nurse was expected to have the confidence to carry out complex orders and procedures, but rarely to question and never to answer back. In other words she learnt through being regularly assessed what was expected of her as a City nurse.

The negative feelings generated by this process were graphically described by two nurses nearing the end of their training. One nurse experienced the ward reports as 'a lot of character bashing'. The other felt that her identity had been crushed.

Yet all these students, whether they felt they were being moulded, seen in a different way to how they saw themselves, having their character bashed or their identity crushed, managed their private feelings in order to behave in the way expected of a City Hospital nurse. The methods by which the students were assessed therefore imposed feeling rules that required emotion work to maintain the image of the City nurse and trained them to stand up in a hierarchical and academically demanding environment.

One tutor observed:

A problem may arise on the ward and the student might get unhappy but they won't say anything to the ward staff because they're frightened of the ward reports.

One student now at the end of training saw the assessments in a more positive and less passive light. She told me that through them she had built up both her confidence and role expectations and in the process learnt from other students to stick up for herself. She said:

You don't think you'll have the confidence and be supportive and help and teach other students. But you build up to teaching and management responsibility through your assessments and you learn from other students to stick up for yourself.

In the final section of this chapter, I examine the way in which the patients portrayed the City nurse in Nightingale's image and the students' reaction to this image.

In Nightingale's image

I observed a classroom discussion during which students were asked to describe the stereotypes patients had of them. They mentioned such images as 'angel', 'beautiful' and 'Florence Nightingale'.

I also found in my interviews with patients that the nurse as angel was a particularly popular image. One patient described a student as an 'angel of mercy' in the context of maintaining composure on a busy night shift when three elderly patients were shouting and confused and wandering up and down the ward. The patient observed that the nurse was almost 'at breaking point and all white faced. I know I couldn't do it. It's hard to hold your temper. But she did very well to cope'. By inference her ability to 'hold her temper' was attributed to her being an 'angel of mercy'.

Associated with the image of the nurse as 'an angel' was also the belief by many patients that nursing was a 'vocation' which required dedication. One patient expressed surprise following discussions with some students because they told her that nursing was a 'job of work'. 'I'd always imagined it was a calling', she said.

The idea that nursing was a vocation epitomised the belief that nurses brought not only natural skills to their chosen occupation, but also deeper qualities of giving and lack of interest in financial reward. Two patients for example, viewed nursing as something 'you've got to have in you'. Another patient saw a nurse's abilities as 'resting so much on the girl, how much she can give to the patient. It goes with that nature that brings them into this sort of vocation'. Another patient reasoned that nursing must be a vocation since nurses 'wouldn't go in it for the money'. These images corresponded with those portrayed in the recruitment posters described in Chapter 1. Nurses had the essential qualifications before they went to school. They were also unlikely to be 'attracted to nursing because of the money'.

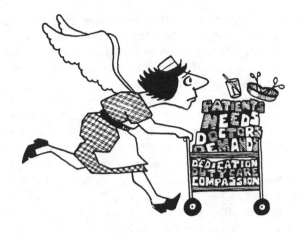

(Source: Cath Jackson)

Nurses resented these images. One student told me that, 'patients call you an angel. I tell them I'm doing it not to go to heaven but as a job. They can't understand that'. A patient who was also a nurse challenged the image of the nurse as 'an angel of mercy'. Anyone can do it (nursing), she said, meaning that you didn't need to have a vocation to be a nurse.

These pictures suggest that, at the level of rhetoric, patients colluded in perpetuating the image of the nurse, a modern day Nightingale, as having 'natural' skills and being vocationally motivated and dedicated. Most students vigorously denied that they had been motivated by a vocation to choose nursing.

In this chapter I have described the sort of people who train as nurses at City Hospital and how their gender, class and ethnic characteristics are associated with the history of the institutions in which they work.

I have also briefly described the methods I used to study the patients, students, nurses and teachers at the City Hospital and school of nursing.

Next I have shown ways in which the Nightingale image of the white, vocationally orientated young woman, is perpetuated at City Hospital through the job prospectus and selection procedures and how continuous assessment trains students to stand up in a hierarchically and academically demanding environment. The ways in which the job prospectus, selection and assessment operate suggest that complex processes are at work. Gender and occupational ideologies shape strategies that may be explained by the emotional labour process of feeling rules and emotion management (Hochschild, 1983).

Examining patients' images of nurses shows how they collude in the perpetuation of the image of the nurse as having 'natural' skills and being vocationally motivated and dedicated. As Oakley (1984) suggests, the qualities of a 'good' woman are closely associated with those of the 'good' nurse. Students vigorously reject the view that they are vocationally motivated to become nurses.

How then are the gender and occupational ideologies described above reflected in the students' plan of training? And how/are nurses formally taught to care?

3 Nothing is really said about care: defining nursing knowledge

Students came to City Hospital with a commitment to care but also to be students in an 'academically demanding' environment. Most of them did not expect that they would so quickly and so soon be counted in the workforce for more than 80 per cent of their training. They were full-time classroom students only 30 out of 156 weeks and a sixth of that was right at the beginning of training in the Foundation Unit. The rest of the time was spent in the wards giving patient care, where they made up two-thirds of the workforce. The experience of finding themselves as principal care givers provoked two reactions. One was that they, the student nurses, were the group of people who cared the most since there were more of them. Secondly, they resented that their learning role was secondary to their role as workers. One student told me angrily, 'You go on the ward. You're not the student nurse at all. You're the workforce and if you learn something then good for you'.

A tutor also observed:

Student nurses don't want to be used as pairs of hands but to have their learning role recognised, that's the problem, and here at City we depend on them as the workforce.

It did not take long before the students began to see the ward and school as two different worlds. Their teachers, who inhabited the airy classrooms and quiet corridors of the school, were rarely seen in the hustle and bustle of the wards. During interviews, students frequently referred to the wards as 'out there'— which symbolised the 'real' world of patients and nurses, doctors and diseases. Sitting in the hushed silence of the comfortable school library surrounded by books, the wards did indeed seem a world away rather than the five-minute walk to the adjacent building.

Often when I walked between the hospital and the school in 'off research' times, I would meet nurses hurrying either on or off duty. They would often stop to fill me in with the most recent events that I had 'missed' on the current ward I was studying. Had I heard that Robin had had another respiratory arrest? Did I know that Peter was going to be transferred to another ward for surgery? Wasn't it terrible that Mr Lawrence had suddenly deteriorated in the night and died? Or the most recent news about the nurses. Lisa passed her assessment, but Mary got a terrible report and is really upset. Then I would arrive at the school minutes later in order to check the timetable to select which class I was going to observe. Titles like 'Passing a Naso-Gastric Tube'; 'The Physiology of the Blood'; or 'How to nurse patients with this or that disease', frequently appeared. Sessions that might have dealt with the feelings around a sudden death, a respiratory emergency or a failed assessment were less easy to identify. Was this why students complained that 'school's got nothing to do with nursing' or that their teachers did not have enough to do with them on the wards, leading them to conclude that: 'It's two different worlds'?

But although the students had minimal contact with the school and their teachers, they experienced their influence at an ideological level throughout training. The school set the 'ideals and standards' of the City nurse and designed the formal content of their training to achieve them.

We saw in the previous chapter that ideologies at City Hospital promoted both the new 'people-orientated' and the old 'biological' approaches to nursing. The selection criteria best illustrated these twin ideologies. On the one hand, students' interest and experience in working with people came as part of their personal and experiential package, whilst on the other, their biological knowledge had to be formally learnt and validated.

As suggested in Chapter 1, national nursing ideologies rejected the image of the nurse as the doctor's assistant based on the medical treatment of disease, in favour of the 'new' nurse committed to care and interpersonal relationships with patients. An alternative knowledge base for nursing was sought which turned away from a biomedical one[1]. The nursing process was identified as a people-orientated philosophy and four-stage work method of assessment, planning, implementation and evaluation, which offered that alternative.

The content of nurse training at City Hospital

Yet despite national ideologies, the theoretical and practical organisation of the three-year programme at City was based on medical specialties, such as paediatrics, obstetrics, geriatrics, gynaecology and psychiatry with the heaviest emphasis being given to four modules each of medical and surgical nursing in the first and final year of training. This in part explained why disease-orientated sessions dominated the timetables.

I was also curious to find out how national and local nursing ideologies were reflected in the curriculum papers given to students at the beginning of training. These papers stated the general course philosophy and the aims, objectives and content of each of the fifteen modules (see Appendix C).

I also wanted to find out whether these ideologies were visible in the classroom by studying the timetables further, observing selected teaching sessions and interviewing teachers and students.

The curriculum papers reflected a dual picture of the new 'people-orientated' and the old 'biological' approaches to nursing. The modular aims and objectives demonstrated a commitment to meeting patients' physical, psychological and social needs, but the suggested content was dominated by the 'natural sciences' in the Foundation Unit and by the signs and symptoms, techniques and procedures associated with medical diagnosis and disease in the subsequent three-year programme.

Given both the academic selection criteria and the suggested content of the Foundation Unit, it is not surprising that students considered secondary school biology to underpin its theoretical content. But they also referred to nursing as working with people and did not necessarily see biology as the natural knowledge base of nursing. One student said, 'It [the Foundation Unit] was very biology-orientated. I thought it would be all practical, which would have been more beneficial'.

Another student described its content 'as all cells and bits that don't connect with the patient'.

They were more likely to describe nursing in terms of the 'basics', i.e. bed-making, bathing, mouth-care, lifting, feeding, toileting, *talking* and *empathy* (my emphasis) with patients. One student proclaimed: 'Nursing isn't a dry boring subject ... we are talking about people'. Another student who believed that 'if people don't matter then you can't do nursing' described care as an essential part of nursing knowledge but was disappointed by its lack of conceptualisation in the curriculum. She said, 'Nothing is really said about care. They [the tutors] say you have to care but nobody actually says what caring is'.

At this early stage of training students still clearly related to the selection criteria that had played an important part in their recruitment to train at City Hospital, i.e. their interest in and experience of working with people.

After six months of training, students talked about knowing 'the basics by now' and needing to know about different techniques and investigations. The knowledge required to nurse was described as 'the solid facts, the diseases, the anatomy and the physiology'.

The students' comments were indicative of a shift in emphasis during the first year away from so-called 'basics' and 'people' work to the 'solid facts' of 'theory' and the techniques and procedures of practice. One student in her third year used Advanced Level biology as a yardstick by which to measure the knowledge and 'absolute facts' that she believed were being 'missed out' in her training programme. She said, ' I did biology up to A level so I do know how much I should know ... I want higher knowledge from the school ... somewhere the absolute facts are being missed out'.

Two other third-year students expressed similar doubts about the state of their knowledge, because they judged it on the basis of its medical and technical content. One of them concluded:

Although you spend a lot of time building up your nursing skills, the depth of knowledge into diseases, drugs and therapy gets rather left by the wayside and I find that my knowledge is really sort of patchy and scanty and there is no sort of depth to it. I've just learnt bits here and there.

This student identified her time on the ward as the place where she built up her nursing skills through practical experience. But she saw these skills as distinct from her 'patchy and scanty' knowledge base which she judged on a biomedical model of 'disease, drugs and therapy'.

Another student described her knowledge as 'fragmented' because she had worked on a number of wards without 'doing any cardiology or seen an appendicectomy' which to her represented the cornerstones of basic medical and surgical nursing experience.

Why then did students shift to judging nursing based on biomedical rather than people-orientated knowledge? One explanation seemed to lie in the way in which their nursing programme was designed around modules based on medical specialties and a curriculum dominated by biomedical knowledge.

Furthermore, the written curriculum also became a reality in the classroom. An analysis of the timetables planned by the nurse tutors showed that the content of their teaching sessions, with the exception of some of the specialties, such as psychiatry, during the second year, closely corresponded with the biomedically orientated curriculum.

During the Foundation Unit and medical modules for example, I found that only 14 per cent of all sessions could be categorised as dealing with a more people-orientated approach to care (see Appendix D). The content of these sessions emphasised such topics as the principles and practice of the nursing process, interpersonal communication, experiential learning, nursing care of patients in pain, and the management of death and dying. I assumed that during these sessions students learnt about the conceptualisation of nursing as care and 'people' work. I chose to observe some of these sessions in order to test my assumption.

Nursing process: philosophy, conceptual device or work method?

First of all, I wanted to find out to what extent the nursing process philosophy and work method was used as a device for conceptualising nursing knowledge and practice as care and 'people' work by both teachers and their students. The evidence provided by the timetables (1 per cent of all sessions) suggested hardly at all. I also attended sessions (only 3 per cent of the total) which fitted in with the underlying conceptual framework of the nursing process such as Henderson's (1960) and Roper's (1976) models for nursing practice based on the activities of daily living[2]. One tutor described these models as 'checklists against which to tick off your knowledge or hang your concepts on'. The way in which the models were taught in the classroom did rather give the impression of a checklist. Students learnt that as nurses, their 'unique function' was to assist patients with up to 14 living activities. These activities covered basic physical, psychological and social needs. The 'checklist' of needs formed the basis for learning how to assess, plan, implement and evaluate patient care following the nursing process format. But the link between the activities of living, patient interviewing to assess their condition and needs, and the planning of appropriate care were not explicitly made. The delay in or lack of 'tie-up' between the conceptual and methodological aspects of the nursing process was expressed by a student at the end of the six-week Foundation Unit. She said:

We learnt a bit about the nursing process but I don't think we realised how important it was. We didn't do a care plan until our last day in school but if the tutors had tied it up with the nursing process and living activities, we would have realised that the two went together. But I didn't realise until then that care plans were part of the nursing process and that was what you did with them.

During interviews with tutors I began to understand why the nursing process did not feature prominently as an integral part of their teaching or as a way of conceptualising nursing. Many of them, for example, interpreted it in different ways. One tutor described the nursing process as about 'feelings and attitudes and more applicable to the ward'. It certainly featured in the curriculum papers in this way, exhorting students to care for patients as people in the module objectives and assessment criteria, but offering very little formal knowledge and guidance on how to do this.

Two tutors who described themselves as 'pro nursing process' were critical of colleagues whose teaching was still 'very task orientated and based on the medical model' or 'not good at equipping students with the necessary communication and interviewing skills'.

Another tutor explained that nurse tutors were having difficulties with the nursing process because of insufficient preparation to use it either in the classroom or ward. Actually, she admitted, 'I do like the medical model and it can be nice and logical and it's scientific and you can do that in school beautifully. I don't think we can throw the medical model out completely because at the end of the day we've got people coming in to hospital with diseases. We've gone overboard thinking it's the person we must look at'.

This tutor's reaction was interesting because she, like many of her colleagues, was finding difficulty conceptualising nursing as people-orientated knowledge. Her view that the medical model can be 'logical' and 'scientific' implied that the nursing process, as an alternative model for conceptualising knowledge, was not.

The group characteristics of the tutors offered some explanation for their difficulties in using the nursing process as a conceptual device. The majority of them had trained and practised as nurses in the pre-nursing process era when the biological view of the nurse's role had been predominant. Furthermore, teacher training programmes were only just beginning to move away from a biomedical model to incorporate more psychology and sociology, in keeping with the nursing process philosophy. More recent thinking suggests that the nursing process is limited as a conceptual device and a number of nursing models have now been proposed to supersede it[3]. These limitations would explain why many of the City tutors had difficulty in using the process as an alternative to bio-medical knowledge.

The students, therefore, had very little reason to view the nursing process as part of the theoretical content of their training, even during the first six months when they clearly related to nursing as people work. To them it was 'a waffly subject that all boils down to common sense in the end' or 'what you do really'. Even though the nursing process offered the potential for identifying and generating people-orientated knowledge, the students did not see it used in this way by their tutors. They began to regard it as 'common sense' and 'what you do' rather than an approach to nursing with its own knowledge base and set of skills.

Like the tutor quoted above, the students saw the nursing process as 'more applicable to the ward' describing it as a work method based on their clinical experiences rather than as classroom abstractions. For example, one student said:

For me the nursing process means patient allocation as opposed to work allocation. It's more thinking of the patient as a whole as opposed to one nurse being responsible for bedpans etc.

The people-orientated approach of the nursing process as work method (patient as opposed to work allocation) was apparent in this description of the nurse *thinking of the patient as a whole* rather than *being responsible for bedpans* (my emphasis).

The ward-based applications and interpretations of the nursing process are discussed in Chapters 5 and 7.

Affective/psychosocial nursing and learning to do emotional labour

The nursing process and associated sessions not only accounted for few classroom sessions on the timetables, but neither did they necessarily offer formal knowledge and guidance to students on nursing as care and people work. This finding fitted in with the student's view that 'nothing is really said about care' within the nurse training programme.

I now turned to the sessions categorised on the timetables as dealing with affective/psychosocial nursing (10 per cent of the total). These sessions covered such topics as interpersonal communication, experiential learning, nursing care of patients in pain and the management of death and dying. I assumed that during these sessions students were most likely to learn about the conceptualisation of nursing as care and people work. I chose to observe some of these sessions in order to find out if this were so, and to see how they related to the notion of training students to do emotional labour. I describe two sessions below, both of which used group discussion as a teaching method.

Patient–nurse perceptions: first-year students

This session was led by a tutor who was a psychiatric nurse specialist. She had specifically been asked to do this session by the general nurse teachers because they believed the topic required psychiatric expertise. Perception was defined at the beginning of the session as 'the interpretations and judgments made by nurses through observation of the way patients behave'. The role and context in which this behaviour took place were discussed.

S(tudent).   Patients don't know how to react to you when you go on to ward wearing your own clothes on your day off.

40

S.   It's the same when you see patients wearing their own clothes, rather than their night things.

T(utor).   Why do you think that is?

S.   Well, what you wear is associated with your role. Wearing night clothes is associated with being a patient, like wearing my uniform is associated with my role as a nurse.

The tutor agrees, then, reflecting on the nurse's role, asks:

Does X (refers to one of the senior teachers by name) still have that thing that you should smile the whole time ?

S.   Yes she still has it.

T.   No wonder patients are confused! [She laughs.]

A student then considers the effects nurses have on patients and says, 'It's dangerous the authority nurses have over patients'.
When she is asked to explain what she means, she replies:

Some patients become 'pets'. We all do it. They're looked at as 'very nice'. Or other patients get the reputation of being an old 'sod' and then you think 'well sister should know her work. If that's her opinion I'd better avoid him'.

S.   Often you find it's not true what they [trained staff] tell you.

S.   We as beginners are very vulnerable and on the side of the patients. Staff nurses have seen it all before and think patients are up to their 'old tricks'.

The content of this session is interesting in terms of its association with learning to do emotional labour. Both nurses and patients were cast in a role symbolised by their respective 'uniforms'. Tutor and students were aware that one of the senior teachers expected them to smile. The importance of smiling as a key 'caring' behaviour was reminiscent of Hochschild's descriptions of emotional labour in the airline industry. Flight attendants were also encouraged to smile by their instructors.
Differences between the two groups of workers (nurses and flight attendants) became apparent, however, as the students described the 'authority' they felt they had over patients. The

hierarchical relationships within the British health care system determined the feeling rules surrounding certain patients. At the beginning of training, students saw themselves as vulnerable and on the side of the patient. But patients could acquire either positive or negative labels which were often legitimised by the trained staff's view of them. Because the students felt that the ward sister 'should know her job' and the staff nurses had seen it all before, they as the juniors should take their cues from them. In the case of the patient who had been labelled an 'old sod' they felt that in order to conform to the rules and reduce internal conflicts they should withdraw their emotional labour by avoiding him.

These strategies were very different from the official ones taught to flight attendants. They also recognised and labelled difficult passengers, but were formally taught to manage anger or irritation through deep acting techniques to enable them to continue their interaction. As the next account illustrates, students at City were expected to learn experientially to induce or suppress feelings irrespective of how they felt about their relationships with patients or colleagues. The classroom sessions gave them the opportunity to describe their emotional work but gave them little knowledge or guidance on how to manage their feelings.

Critical incidents: third-year students

The use of critical incidents (Clamp, 1980) as a teaching method was popular with the nurse teachers during the third year of training[4]. The purpose of the method was to encourage students in small group sessions, led by a tutor, to draw on incidents from their ward work in order to learn about their feelings, behaviour and attitudes.

One tutor described the method in the following way:

If you control the discussion firmly enough without being seen to control it then you can pick out the things that you actually ought to draw attention to, the things that can be learnt from. The students have a variety and richness of experience to offer. They might start out thinking it's a grouse session but if you can you get them to the point that they can see they are learning.

The tutor realised that the students had difficulties in recognising that they were learning from their experiences in this apparently circuitous way rather than from the more familiar didactic classroom situation of being systematically taught formal knowledge about a clearly defined topic.

One student, for example, gave a mixed reaction to a critical incident session at which we had both been present. 'All we are doing is as a group of friends having conversations' (implying that the session wasn't a 'real' teaching session). She goes on to show some insight that because the 'conversations' are formalised through the lesson title 'Critical incidents', participants, especially the shy ones, are given permission to mention things they normally wouldn't. The student is also aware that the feeling within the group is important. She concludes: 'They will say it to their friends, just because their expression is enough to help support them because they understand'.

During the session, students did indeed describe a range of feelings whilst in contact with patients, feelings such as *fear* (because an aggressive patient on night duty threatened to throw his bed at them), *failure* (at being unable to cope personally with an offensive patient) or *guilt* at escorting an abusive, uncooperative patient home from hospital and persuading his desperate relatives to take him back. The students received both peer group support and empathy during the session, because many could identify similar emotionally demanding situations. But the way in which they expressed their feelings suggested that support in retrospect was too late: they had needed it at the time, when the labour of maintaining an outward appearance of calm and competence had cost them emotionally dear.

We take up the story of the student who felt guilty for persuading relatives to accept a desperately disturbed patient home from an acute surgical ward in a bid to have him admitted to a psychiatric hospital. The plan had been thought up by doctors and delegated by the trained staff to two third-year students. It was discovered some days later that the patient was still at home.

Discussing the session with me in an interview later that same day, the student who had given a mixed reaction to 'Critical incidents' as a teaching method used the incident of the disturbed patient to comment further on its limitations. She said:

43

I was amazed at that incident, where Belle took that bloke home. I was almost speechless, because anyone who's a student nurse can understand.

PS. What do you mean ?

S. Well the tutor just called it 'unfortunate, an unfortunate situation to be in'. Unfortunate! That girl was still screwed up about what she might have done to the emotional side of the sister of that bloke and she brought it up in a lecture and she wasn't supported.

PS. I thought the tutor was quite supportive.

S. How could she be? It was a conversation. Belle thought that because she said it out loud she could be supported. It's not enough to say 'Well it's the medical and trained staff's problem because it was their decision to send him home. You're not guilty. Don't feel guilty'. How can you not feel guilty! She knew that she shouldn't have taken him home. She was the one who in the end had to convince that woman to take her brother into a home that was falling apart. She was the one who made the promises to the woman that her brother would soon be transferred to the psychiatric hospital. She was the one who made the longstanding arrangements. I just felt so much for her. I thought 'Where were you when you found out that man was still at home?' Were you standing at the phone, or sitting at report and staff nurse just passed it on to you as a bit of gossip and your heart sank because you knew you were the one who had promised his sister?

I felt humbled as the student poured out her feelings. I reflected that I might very easily have reacted like the tutor because I had not grasped the full impact and implications of the incident as seen by this student nurse. I knew that the student who had been involved in the incident appeared very distressed as she described what had happened, and it is likely that the tutor arranged to see her to talk about it after the session.

The student continued:

S. I don't know if you heard me, but I asked who went in that ambulance. Two student nurses. That is appalling! Some doctor has said that it is the only way to get somebody out of hospital and has made his decision and wiped his hands of the situation

44

and it went down until it could go down no further. And what was that student told when she left that ward? 'We have a lot to thank you for'. They should be doing more than thanking her. She will probably have that memory always.

This vivid account of the feelings generated in one student by the recounting of a critical incident showed the potential power of the method in offering students insights into emotional labour and the management of feelings on the wards. It also shows the need for systematic follow-up by teachers of some incidents and the need for careful contact with students and staff on the wards to be available to offer support closer to when such incidents occur. It also demonstrates the way in which the hierarchical structure of the hospital allowed emotional labour to be withdrawn by senior staff, especially doctors 'who wiped their hands of the situation', and deflected downwards to the juniors. The role of hierarchy in shaping emotional labour is discussed further in Chapter 7.

The psychiatric nursing module

In the second year of training, students undertook specialist modules, designed to give them a variety of experiences other than general medical and surgical nursing. These modules included placements on a number of specialist wards such as obstetrics, paediatrics, care of the elderly and psychiatry. For many students their second year represented a period away from what they saw as mainstream nursing, but others enjoyed the exposure to different types of patients and work priorities.

The psychiatric nursing module, coming at the end of the second year, was singled out as being of particular significance. The aims of the module clearly articulated nursing as people work prioritising patients' psychological and social needs and identifying student needs in terms of emotional support. One tutor thought that the module emphasised the students' personal development more than at any other time of their training. She said:

There is something about the whole atmosphere of the psychiatric hospital which seems particularly good for them. It's the fact that someone values them as a person. Someone values their contribution, listens to what they say. It is so different from anything they've come across before. I think they get a lot of time and attention.

A student described the experience as teaching her 'a lot about the importance of talking to your patients and that sort of psychological side of their care. I think you are much more aware of it'.

The psychiatric module exposed students to an alternative knowledge base which was psychological and sociological in nature and translated into interpersonal and interviewing skills associated with people work. However, the module only lasted 9 weeks, and unless the students returned to environments which valued the 'psychological side of care' they quickly readjusted to a biomedical view of nursing[5].

Informal training for people work: feeling rules and emotion management

The psychiatric nursing module was too short to convince the majority of the students that they learnt their communication skills in any way other than informally. The most common examples given were those of role modelling and ward-based experience, and certainly not from classroom teaching or discussion.

First-year students told me:

You saw sister or staff nurse in some tricky situations with patients. They handled them so well. You *just* learnt by watching how they talked to them.

Or:

You see how the nurses sort of manage patients and talk to them and you *just* pick things up. It's *just* their general attitude; you think 'that's a really nice way to treat someone' ... and they show an example.

And again:

I think you *just* learn by watching the way other people do things, like talking to dying patients.

46

Another student described communication skills as something she learnt through exposure to difficult situations during patient contact i.e. *'just* through experience'.

It comes with practice anyway. The more you come in contact with patients in difficult situations you learn how to cope because that's how the third years have learnt ... *just* through experience.

The point about all these comments is that the students might be seen to minimise the learning of emotional care by the repeated use of *'just* learning; *'just* picking it up'; *'just* by watching'; *'just* through experience'. An alternative explanation is that they apply the meaning of 'just' to these activities to infer the 'naturalness' of such learning as opposed to formal classroom teaching. The danger here is that the skills acquired through these activities might also be regarded as 'natural' and not requiring any or much skill to perform or effort to acquire[6].

A student who had recently taken her state final examination said that she also learnt by watching other people and identifying 'a good model', but she went beyond the actual experience to reflecting on its content. She said:

You think 'I'll remember that' or 'that's not the way I'd do it'. Then again it's almost inspirational or off the cuff. You think 'I've never met this before; I've got to act'. Or you go off duty and think how you've handled something and sift through it.

As well as role modelling, she also described a form of unconscious or semi-conscious 'acting' in which she responded to new situations and then reflected upon them when she went off duty. In this way she was able to incorporate behaviours and responses in her future repertoires of emotion management. By watching and reflecting she was able to 'know immediately that's wrong, and from then on you're better at it yourself because you know what you should do'.

The other students were more typical in that they did not describe any cognitive process through which they learnt to manage their emotions, but believed that they would learn 'just' through exposure to examples and models of good care.

The minimisation of learning to respond to patients' emotional needs was also reflected in the belief that students brought with them the character and qualities to be able to care.

A first-year student said:

You have to be, even as a first warder, to have the character to be able to talk to strangers, and very quickly. If you haven't got that then I don't think you can nurse well.
   I think that if you're basically a caring person, which presumably you are if you come in to nursing, then I think you have your own sort of procedure. I don't think you should try and make everyone the 'standard' nurse.

Thus the students, just like their recruiters in Chapter 2, saw being a 'caring person' or 'able to talk to strangers' as part of the package that you brought with you as a nurse, not skills that had to be learnt and sustained. Teaching communication skills was seen by this last nurse, and by many of her colleagues, as taking away her personal communication style and replacing it with a 'standard' set of procedures[7].
   Two other students at the beginning and end of training described expectations to be 'nice' to all patients. But they also recognised that there were circumstances under which they could not sustain one of the key characteristics of the City nurse, the capacity to remain 'on an even keel'.
   The first-year student felt pressure to be 'nice' to patients. But she was quite clear that she would only be 'nice' to patients if as part of the equal exchange of 'niceness', they were also 'nice' to her. She said:

I'll never say I particularly like all the patients. You're told you've got to be nice to them but I don't think you have to be if they're not being nice to you.

This student was typical of the City nurse in that she came from a middle-class family. Her father was a company director and her mother a teacher. But she came from a part of the country that had a reputation for 'plain speaking'. She spoke with a strong regional accent and gained a reputation for 'bluntness'. When I interviewed her, she was just coming to terms with the City Hospital expectations and deciding whether or not she wanted to 'learn the rules'.
   The student who had recently completed her training said:

There are times when you're tired, you do and say things you wouldn't normally do. I remember the first time I snapped at

48

a patient, I felt mortified, as I thought that nurses never show that they are personally hurt. Now I don't take that view.

The student identified 'when you're tired' as a time when she might 'do and say things' that weren't 'normal'. In other words she was describing conditions under which she could no longer induce or suppress her own feelings in deference to the patient's. She had found this a liberating experience, in that she was able to acknowledge to herself that she had feelings that mattered. I wondered what might have been special about her personal biography that had allowed her to move from feeling 'mortified' to recognising that she had a right to feel 'personally hurt'. She was older than the majority of City students when she started training, having first obtained a degree in history. She also expressed a keen interest in people, their motivations and behaviours, and later went on to do a postgraduate qualification in psychiatric nursing.

Learning to communicate and emotion management: patients' views

The patients that I interviewed fell somewhere in between the view that nurses had to have certain qualities to be able to communicate with others, but also that part of their training should strengthen those qualities. A selection of comments that illustrate this point are presented below:

The nurse has got to know her 'nursing' but the training must be right. Then it's her humanity immediately after that.

You probably can't teach them to communicate, but you can advise them and if aspects of their personality will respond, you can teach them certain functions and give them hints and aids to guide them along those lines.

It's got to be there [the ability to communicate] although I think you can mould it.

Thus the nurse had to have: humanity, but her training had to be right; the type of personality that would respond to guidance; or an innate ability to communicate, which could then be

49

moulded. The use of the word 'mould' was reminiscent of the student who felt that she was being moulded as a 'City type'.

There were also those patients who gave a sense that the students were being trained to manage their emotions.

You need to train nurses to care for people and not to panic.

It's part of the training to learn to put up with a lot when dealing with old people. They can be cantankerous and the nurses need a lot of patience to hold it back.

Thus the nurse had to learn to care, but not to panic, and also to put up with a lot.

In summary, the formal knowledge base of the nurse training programme at City Hospital was biomedical, but the informal knowledge base promoted a people-orientated approach to care in keeping with national ideologies. The national ideology looked for formalisation of people-orientated knowledge and recognition of the nurse's unique skills, distinct from that of medicine's. At City, the local ideology promoted care as part of the 'natural' package of the nurse brought by virtue of the caring, female qualities that brought her into nursing. The local ideology was reinforced by informal knowledge and ward experience, rather than by looking at care as something that needs to be formally taught, supported and learnt.

The reason why 'nothing is really said about care' by the nurse teachers seemed to be because many of them either had doubts whether, or were unsure how, the content and teaching of nursing knowledge should differ from its traditional bio-medical base. Few of them therefore used the nursing process as a conceptual means to defining an alternative approach to nursing knowledge from a biomedical one.

During sessions designated as affective/psychosocial nursing, teachers recognised the need and attempted to train students to care emotionally for patients as distinct from carrying out technical and physical tasks based on a biomedical approach to nursing. But these sessions were limited both in quantity and quality. They gave the students an occasional opportunity to describe their emotional work, but little knowledge or guidance on how to manage their feelings.

The students' own view, in the absence of an alternative model provided by their teachers, was that emotional care could not be formally taught. The psychiatric module coming at the end of their second year gave them all too brief a glimpse of an alternative perspective.

Patients held the view that, whilst nurses brought innate qualities essential to nursing, they also required training to strengthen them. Some patients and students also recognised that emotion management was required to induce and suppress feelings to maintain an outward appearance of calm.

My conclusion was that, at City Hospital, nursing continued to be seen as women's natural work, devalued and de-skilled because it drew its status and prestige from biomedical knowledge associated with medical techniques and procedures which treated diseases rather than people.

How then was nursing perceived from the point of view of practice, in the 'different world' of the ward?

4 You learn from what's wrong with the patient: defining nursing work

In the 'different world' of the ward, students moved through 15 clinical placements according to the medical specialties that also defined the formal content of their training[1]. At the City Hospital, as in most British teaching hospitals, the wards acquired their labels according to the specialty of the consultant physicians and surgeons who worked there, treating patients and teaching medical students. The wards were roughly divided between medicine and surgery, and then subdivided according to such specialties as oncology, neurology, gastroenterology, cardiology or orthopaedics. Specialties such as geriatrics, psychiatry, paediatrics, obstetrics and gynaecology were likely to be on separate wards and even in separate 'sister' hospitals. As the students progressed through their 15 placements, they not only changed wards but in some instances also hospitals, in order to fulfil their medically defined training requirements. The reason why they continued to see nursing as a branch of medicine thus became apparent.

One student summed up this view when she reacted to the idea that all ward experiences irrespective of medical specialty were of equal value because 'it's all nursing. I think it's very blind of anybody to believe that', she said, 'because you learn from what's *wrong* with the patient'. In other words nursing for this student, like the majority of her colleagues, depended on the medical diagnosis of the patient and by association the medical specialty of the ward.

You learn from what's wrong with the patient: how medical specialties legitimise nursing work

In this section I explore further why the student reacted negatively to the idea that all ward experiences were of equal value because 'it's all nursing'.

As I talked to other students about their clinical experiences the more it became apparent that a pecking order of ward specialties existed[2]. This pecking order was not unique to the students but reflected a common societal view that valued high-tech medicine and marginalised the caretaking activities associated with caring for the elderly and chronically sick. It was also in direct contradiction with national nursing ideologies, which wanted to de-link nursing from medicine. The pecking order also reflected the role confusion experienced by students as both workers and learners. Since their formal knowledge and practice was based on medical specialties, the prestige and status afforded to certain of those specialties shaped the way in which they defined the content of their work and learning and its physical, technical or emotional components and not national nursing ideologies. The pecking order also reflected the students' shift from people-orientated nursing to a biomedical approach, described in the previous chapter. These findings are hardly surprising, but what they do show us is that the new forms of nurse training promoted by the national training bodies were not sufficiently established to counter this divide[3].

The general medical wards were lowest in the pecking order. Many of the patients were elderly and suffering from chronic conditions. Then there were the specialist medical wards such as neurology, cardiology and oncology. Thirdly, there were the surgical wards where 'you learn a completely different type of nursing from medicine, because you have to be more alert'.

At the bottom were the general medical wards where the content of the work was characterised as mostly physical. At the top were the surgical wards where the work was seen as mostly technical. In between were the specialist medical wards where the work was identified as both technical and physical and in the case of oncology, also emotional.

The psychiatric experience, coming at the end of their second year of specialties, was different from anything else the nurses experienced elsewhere in their training, because the content of their work and learning was defined only in emotional terms.

Students held low opinions about the value of their learning on some general medical wards. One student went so far as to compare it to working in a nursing home before she started training, commenting that 'I don't think I've learnt a lot more on the medical wards than I did when I was working in the nursing home'. Her judgement was based on the amount of physical care that patients required according to their age and general

53

medical condition rather than the technical procedures required by surgical patients.

Caring for elderly patients was seen by students as *'just having to help old people get up in the morning, get dressed and persevere with them'*. Other students spoke disparagingly of elderly patients who had been admitted to the general wards for 'social' rather than 'medical' problems. A problem was defined as 'social' if patients could no longer care for themselves because of impaired function due to ageing and chronic rather than acute disease. Such patients were described as 'bed blockers', as taking up valuable space from patients in need of 'real' medical and nursing attention[4].

Three general female wards were constantly cited by students as being at the bottom of the pecking order of medical specialties (and hence of learning potential), because they admitted a high percentage of elderly patients who fell into this category. The wards were described as 'heavy' because of the high physical dependency of many of the patients. At best, these wards were seen as offering 'brilliant learning experience' for first-year students because of the 'good basic experience' they offered.

In my questionnaire survey of the learning environment amongst first- and third-year students on 12 specialist and general medical wards at City Hospital (see Appendix E), only 10 per cent of comments identified care of the elderly, 'heavy', 'basic' or 'routine' work as valuable to learning. These students were almost exclusively first-years. A further 21 per cent of comments on work and other experiences which they saw as least valuable to learning identified routine/basic work generated by elderly and/or physically dependent patients. Respondents were just as likely to be first- as third-year students. Thus, although the majority of students who identified basic routine work as valuable to learning were first-years, not all of them shared the same view.

Overall, as Tables E3 and E5 in Appendix E illustrate, technical nursing and medical knowledge, investigations and treatment were more likely to be identified by students as valuable to their learning than any other category of ward experience.

Students learnt very quickly to distinguish between the work of general and specialist medical wards. For example, one student, less than six months into training, compared the 'heavy' routine work of her first allocation to the specialist neurological ward where she was now assigned. 'It's unlike most other medical wards' she said in a thrilled voice 'because there are loads of different illnesses and multiple sclerosis and all that and people coming in for tests and lumbar punctures and things'. In her excitement she saw neurology as exotic diseases and tests rather than uncertainty, unpleasant symptoms and long-term suffering for patients and their families.

Experience on surgical wards was predominantly seen as learning about techniques: patients were much more likely to have intravenous infusions, urinary catheters, surgical dressings, suction and other types of surgical drainage than their counterparts on the medical wards. On the surgical wards, there were a variety of techniques that students could observe being performed: changing dressings or intravenous infusion bags, inserting catheters, or removing surgical drains and stitches. As one student observed: 'You can learn from watching techniques being done'. Another student was excited by learning to care for surgical patients with a very quick turnover, and to manage emergencies such as plummeting blood pressures or haemorrhaging wounds.

Recognising emotion work

The oncology wards were the only wards in the students' 'general' experience where the nature of their work and associated learning was unequivocally described as having an explicit emotional component. One reason for this was the medical legitimisation of emotion work within the specialty[5]. One student described how it 'began to dawn' on her when she was on an oncology ward at the end of her first year 'the amount of psychological needs that people have'. 'Until then' she said 'I hadn't realised what people's needs are when they are in hospital'. Another student described the oncology ward as the place where she learnt about 'human emotion', because 'you see the patients in such a lot of trouble'. She also described the work in terms of oncological techniques and specialist nursing. The medical legitimisation of emotion work within oncology was reinforced by the powerful image of cancer in society as a symbol of suffering and death, vividly described by Susan Sontag (1983) in her essay on 'Illness as Metaphor'.

I was interested by another student's perspectives, which illustrated how a medical specialty served to legitimise nursing's

55

emotional as well as technical components by comparing her experiences on an ophthalmology with an oncology ward. She said of the ophthalmology ward:

I would have liked to have been taught more about 'the eyes' really on that ward. I mean it's quite fun chatting to the patients but the actual nursing is boring. Anybody can bathe an eye. But I dare say if you are an ophthalmologist in a clinic it's different. It's more a doctor's thing than a nurse's from my point of view.

I then asked her what she thought of as a 'nurse's thing'. She replied: 'Maybe oncology is much more of a nurse's world because there is so much more psychological care'.

In other words, this student perceived oncology patients as generating 'psychological care' as part of the work, whereas patients with eye problems were merely 'quite fun' to chat to.

On the other hand, this student also suggests that psychological care associated with oncology, is more a 'nurse's world' than a specialty (i.e. ophthalmology) which she sees as being more dependent on medical skills.

Yet in the ward survey, only 15 per cent of comments (Table E4 in Appendix E) identified the emotional components of nursing (e.g. care of terminal patients and their relatives, talking to them and controlling their pain) as valuable to learning. Students were more likely to identify these experiences when they were allocated to oncology wards, even though patients on all medical wards might be in pain, suffer from cancer, die or need nurses to talk to.

We have already observed in the previous chapter the importance of the psychiatric nursing module for making students more aware of the 'psychological side' of patient care. One student described the mechanisms used on a psychiatric ward to focus on the emotional aspects of the work. She described what happened when feelings ran high for both patients and staff.

If there was an intense staff interaction, say when the patient's being very aggressive and you get upset. It would be put directly to someone in charge. Everything would stop. There would be a discussion. It wouldn't just be 'what should we do about this?' First of all the trained staff would start on you. 'How does this upset you? Are you sure you feel alright?

56

This plan of action isn't working with this patient. Let's go and talk to them and let them know'.

The focus of work on the psychiatric ward was clearly defined around relationships and feelings and how to manage them systematically. The person in charge would stop 'everything' to discuss a patient care issue and how it affected the nurses. This approach was very much in contrast to most general wards, where (with the possible exception of oncology) patient care was organised to 'keep going' in order to manage high turnover, technical procedures and 'heavy' physical work, irrespective of how the students felt. But the urgency of the work, and the power and persuasiveness of the image of acute hospital nursing, was not only felt by students. A committed psychiatric nurse and teacher told me that, even after years of working in a psychiatric hospital, she still experienced a fleeting feeling on entering the corridors of City, busy with nurses and porters escorting patients on trolleys and wheelchairs and intravenous drips, that this was 'real' nursing and not the emotional labour of the psychiatric wards.

When the feelings don't fit

Survey findings showed that the nature of the work on all 12 medical wards generated a range of feelings in students which could have been appropriately handled using the approach described by the student allocated to the psychiatric ward. The students were asked to rate their feelings of stress or anxiety whilst on a ward on a four-point scale from 3.0 (frequently experienced) to 0 (never experienced) during their eight-week allocation. The average scores for the 12 wards ranged from 2.24 to 1.44 (see Table E6(a), Appendix E). No ward achieved a 'zero' stress rating, i.e. anxiety or stress was 'never' not experienced by students as a group on any one ward. Four wards were shown to have high stress ratings that were statistically significant compared with the others (see Table E6(b), Appendix E). Two of these wards were oncology wards, and the other two had very demanding workloads for different reasons. One ward was a 'heavy' female medical ward with low staffing levels, and the other was a male medical ward with a high turnover of acutely ill patients.

Students were also asked to comment on the causes of stress and anxiety on the wards. The nature and volume of the work, ward specialty, type of patients and low staffing levels were frequently implicated. For example, one student found the specialty of oncology 'imposed stress on me as a person' whilst another student experienced stress, physical tiredness and depression because of feeling unable to get the work done on a 'heavy female medical ward'. She implied that her feelings were partly to do with the type of work generated by dependent elderly female patients, but also the lack of staff to carry out the work. Dying patients were mentioned as causes of stress particularly on the oncology wards, but also on two other wards (gastroenterology and cardiology). Fear of patients suffering from cardiac arrests created stress and anxiety for students on the two cardiology wards, even though such incidents rarely happened.

Students also expressed feelings about self and work (or colleagues) as a secondary cause of stress and anxiety. The students said they experienced the following feelings about themselves: inadequate, unsure and defensive, often because they felt unsupported by the trained staff. On one ward a student attributed feelings of 'annoyance and frustration' to 'hierarchical and unfriendly' staff relations.

Common feelings on the heavy female medical wards were boredom, frustration and guilt, associated with the type of patients who required a lot of physical care with low learning value in the students' eyes, but also insuffcient time and staffing to get through the work. A first-year student at the end of her allocation to one of these wards felt 'overworked and very tired'.

But students still rated patient care as being good on these wards (see Table E7 in Appendix E). These scores were amongst the most favourable. The findings suggest two things: firstly, that students, as the principal care givers, were rating their own care and secondly that, despite understaffing and high patient workloads, they felt they were giving patients good care. This assumption further suggests that students laboured both physically and emotionally to care for the patients by suppressing their own feelings.

A third-year student who found patients frustrating was working on an oncology ward. She explained that she did not really want to be allocated to this ward, because her mother had died of cancer. The student found the female oncology patients 'frustrating and often unwilling to help themselves'. The comment suggests that little attention was paid to this student's individual needs, since neither the trained nor the tutorial staff appeared to be aware of her particular situation and/or feelings related to her mother's death. It is also possible that the student did not feel able to tell anyone how she was feeling, because of the need to be seen to cope. Her feelings of frustration at nursing patients with cancer, the disease which had killed her mother, were transmitted through her words. It was even possible that somewhere in her subconscious she felt that her mother had also been unwilling to help herself, but that she also felt frustrated at being unable to help her.

That the students felt deeply about themselves, the patients and their work is apparent in all these descriptions. But the way in which the work was defined according to medical criteria set the feeling rules of the general wards, which in turn determined that the students kept their feelings to themselves.

Even an oncology ward could not accommodate the range of feelings experienced by students, especially when they related to their personal histories. When feelings were not legitimised by the feeling rules of the ward, the students felt stressed or anxious for feeling them. They therefore engaged in emotion work to present a different emotional self in the public arena of the ward.

These findings, like the account of the critical incident described in the previous chapter, show us how students frequently found themselves in emotionally charged situations. These situations went beyond the medical and technical definitions of their training and back to nursing as people work. This was reflected in the way in which students used patients' personal characteristics as well as what was 'wrong' with them as a way of describing their work and learning.

One student, who clearly recognised that nursing work went beyond the boundaries of medical specialties, described the wards at City Hospital as being 'so keyed up to a certain specialty, not nursing care-wise but the doctors who are orientated in that way. That's what they're good at and that's what they deal with. And when you get a patient who isn't their sort of norm then they do tend to be at a bit of a loss'. We can postulate that when the doctors 'are at a bit of a loss' it is then that they 'dump' patients on nurses.

We have already seen one example of this in the critical incident account where a student nurse found herself carrying out a plan 'thought up by the doctors' to get a patient who wasn't 'their sort of norm' into a psychiatric hospital.

We also saw that the students received limited formal training or support to deal with such emotionally charged situations, and few classroom or ward discussions gave them the opportunity to discuss their feelings systematically, both the positive and negative things which they felt about themselves and their patients.

It is not surprising, therefore, that there were certain types of patients that students preferred to nurse to others, and 'liking' someone not only facilitated good interpersonal relationships but also helped their learning. As one student put it: 'You learn from the patients and you adapt to their different characters, especially the patients you like the best'.

This view of 'liking' the patient links up with student perspectives on 'being nice to patients'. Students previously quoted in Chapter 2 recognised that, although they were expected to 'be nice' to everyone, there were certain conditions under which this was not possible. They expected reciprocity from patients. This view was expressed about Mr Bear, an elderly patient who had recently been discharged home. A student recalled: 'Mr Bear looked so happy when he was discharged. He was very grateful and so easy to nurse; he was a lovely man. His wife said "He always said to me how good you nurses were" '. Investing emotional labour was clearly easier with 'grateful' patients like the 'lovely' Mr Bear[6].

There are some patients you'd rather nurse than others: issues of age, gender and race

I concluded that the wards at the bottom of the students' pecking order of 'good' nursing experience admitted a high percentage of elderly female patients with general medical conditions. These patients were rated as generating a high physical workload with poor learning potential.

One student said that one of the reasons why she preferred nursing younger patients (i.e. people in their thirties and forties) was that she found she had a lot more consideration for their feelings. I suppose you shouldn't have, she added guiltily, but you've got to do so much more for the elderly than for younger patients. By this she meant that the physical demands of working with the elderly left little time for considering their individual feelings. But she also felt that she had more in common with patients in their thirties than patients of her grandparents' generation.

Part of the reason for the unpopularity of elderly women patients was because their toileting requirements were seen to generate such physically demanding work. Elderly men could use urinals either sitting in a chair or lying in bed. The urinals were kept in a wire hanger on the side of their beds, so many of them could help themselves when necessary.

However, elderly women had to be helped on to bedpans or commodes which were stored in the sluice. Each time they wanted to use the bedpan or commode they had to ring for the nurse. She then had to help the patient to the bathroom or bring the commode or the bedpan to the bedside. The curtains then had to be drawn and the patient helped on to either. When the patient was ready she was helped off and made comfortable. All this took a lot of time, especially if up to ten patients on a ward needed to be assisted in this way.

It is interesting that patients frequently commented on the 'endless patience' students had 'with the old ones'. Knowing as I did how negatively students often felt about nursing elderly patients, this suggested that they worked on these negative feelings to appear as if they had 'endless patience'.

Students' views on patients' gender were not only related to the physical component of their work, but also their social relations. Many of their expectations and interpretations were based on gender stereotypes. For example, two students on the eve of their first ward allocation thought they would prefer working with men because:

Women are fussy. They expect a 'hotel service' as if they were on holiday. Men are more considerate of nurses. They've got more pride to get on their feet and they don't like women doing things.

Another student, also at the beginning of training, thought it would be easier to work on a men's ward:

Because they are more encouraging than women and they like being fussed over. Women don't. They feel their indepen-

61

dence has gone as mothers and they say 'You should be able to do it [nursing work] better'.

Following her first ward experience of nursing women, this student thought that her predictions had been confirmed:

I think that men would be more grateful. A lot of the women like to be independent. They don't like you telling them what to do. They say 'I could teach you nurses a few things'. Some of them expect you to do everything and they don't say 'please' and 'thank you'.

Another student thought that women 'called out for you. Men are more sort of passive and far more independent'.

These comments show the issue of nursing as women's work. Female patients as wives and mothers were seen as having some expertise in the type of activities that nurses undertook, the tasks described as women's attributes (Ungerson, 1983b). Nurses felt threatened but also resented having to do things for female patients which the patients, as women, usually did for others. They were harder on the women because of this, and expected more gratitude from them. They also expected women to 'take advantage' of their stay in hospital by seeing it as time off from their domestic tasks. Many nurses also expected that, because of this, women patients would also 'take advantage' of them.

The effects of gender on nurse–patient relationships in long-stay geriatric hospitals are discussed by Evers (1981b). She suggested that the 'mothering' model adopted by many of the nurses in caring for their elderly patients in her study was more suited to male patients, since men are used to being serviced in their domestic lives by women. Women, on the other hand, were not used to being serviced by anybody and wanted to maintain their independence.

Although I found in my study that the outcome was similar, the students did not articulate their role as a 'mothering' one, but associated their 'non-technical' activities with the basic skills they acquired in their first few weeks of nursing. Their emotional work was part of the package they brought with them as white middle-class women, which included a range of gender stereotypes which shaped their relationships with male and female patients.

A third-year student preferred nursing men for the following reasons:

> I just find men easier to talk to a lot of the time and they have got a different idea of hospitals. Women can almost expect to be waited on as if they've come in for a rest. Men want to get out of hospital as quickly as possible and they just want to be as independent as possible.

Other students found women easier to talk to because of being women. One nurse found that women were 'more open to discussion' whereas 'men see you just as a nurse'. Another student preferred nursing women because she thought that 'old men touch you up'.

One of the few male interviewees had the following views on nursing male and female patients:

> Patients react differently to male nurses. Women appreciate having a man about the place. It's just a change in atmosphere perhaps. You look upon the technicalities in much the same way, like dressings and getting your drips through on time. In the more social aspects I think probably women talk more easily to women. I think perhaps men talk more easily to women as well, although I think it varies a lot.

These comments illustrate that nurses recognised that gender was important in terms of their social relations and ability to talk with each other. Sexuality was only alluded to and requires further exploration. However, students talked at some length about dealing with violent patients, usually men, and the underlying sexuality implicit in their accounts emerged. The accounts provide further evidence of the lack of opportunity to discuss their feelings systematically, both positive and negative, which they felt about themselves and their patients and how to handle them.

When emotional labour is the work: the case of violent patients

Tracy, a student at the end of her allocation to the ward with the highest stress/anxiety rating of all 12 medical wards, was in a low physical and emotional state when I interviewed her. She was losing her voice because of a severe respiratory infection. Many of the nurses had been sick, she said, which she put down to the stressful conditions on the ward.

I had worked on that ward a few months prior to the interview. The workload was unpredictable because the physicians admitted many of their patients from the hospital's accident and emergency department. Being in the centre of the inner city, many of the patients who were admitted were young men who were drug users and who had overdosed. Apart from their precarious medical conditions in the initial stages of their admission, they could be complicated people to relate to: charming, manipulative and needing their drugs. Part of their rehabilitation was to try to convince them that they needed to be referred to a drug treatment centre. The nurses were on the front line, negotiating the doctors' instructions with the patients. A number of factors affected these negotiations, not least that the nurses and patients were part of the same generation.

Tracy described to me how one such patient who had been on the ward during her allocation had created a lot of stress for her personally. Having recovered from his overdose, the patient, who was over six feet tall, wandered about the ward clad only in his underpants. 'I found this behaviour very sexually suggestive and potentially violent', she said, 'I think partly because of his size. After all I'm only five foot and he towered over me.'

She explained that the doctors offered the patient psychiatric help, but he refused it. After that she said, 'they kept away from him as much as possible. In the end I couldn't go near him either'. Tracy was very upset that she had felt this way, and was unable to justify her withdrawal, even though the doctors had 'kept away from him' also. 'I learnt something about myself she said – I felt I had failed. Never before did I realise that there were certain patients I just couldn't cope with'.

Like the good woman and nurse that she was, Tracy, until this point in her training (the middle of her third year), expected to cope with all patients and types of behaviours. Even though she had felt frightened and threatened, she still expected to induce or suppress her feelings in order to maintain an outward appearance of calm rather than withdraw from the situation. The realisation that there were limits filled her with a sense of failure. Even though doctors might choose to withdraw from the situation, she still believed that nurses shouldn't.

While I was a participant observer on another ward, I observed another student, Mary, confronting a similar situation. The patient in question was Jay, a man in his forties, admitted with episodes of confusion, aggression and violent outbursts. The cause was unclear. He was a professional soldier and there was a suggestion that his behaviour was a reaction to the stress of being in a war zone. He was tall and good-looking and looked every inch the part of a hero in a war film. But there the stereotypical gallantry ended. He would wander off the ward, and any attempts at restraint precipitated aggressive and threatening behaviour. He was particularly confused at night. Two student nurses, 21 years old, were expected to take charge of Jay, along with 20 other patients at least six of whom were acutely ill. On the last night of a seven night stretch, Mary reported sick. The staff nurse told me she was not surprised. 'I heard Mary talking to Jay this morning', she said, 'and her voice was cracking'.

When Mary came back the following week she told me how upset she'd felt over Jay's behaviour. 'We had a lot of sick patients', she said, 'and yet we had to watch that Jay didn't wander off the ward during the night. And you were never sure how he might react to you. We had absolutely no help from the doctors, although the night sisters were quite supportive. I wanted to say to Jay "Look here mate stop messing about" but I felt that I couldn't'.

When I asked her why that was, she said that it was because that was not the way one was expected to talk to patients, irrespective of how you felt. Besides, she didn't know how Jay would react.

For Mary, like Tracy, the costs were high of maintaining emotional labour when confronted by a potentially violent young male patient. Tracy withdrew her labour by avoiding the patient, but felt she had failed. Mary supressed feelings of what she really wanted to say to the patient, but reported sick, the strain having been heard in her voice by a staff nurse on the previous shift.

Dispelling the stereotypes: issues of race

Students described their preference for nursing certain patients based on age and gender stereotypes, but not race. It would not have been acceptable for the City type of nurse (i.e. white and middle-class) in the 'service of others' to express racial prejudice publicly. Whilst I was a participant observer, however, I found that racial stereotypes emerged as an important issue from time to time in a predominantly white middle-class environment. The City Hospital was located in the inner city, with an ethnically diverse population. The majority of patients admitted to the hospital, however, were referred from outside the district. Most of them were white and middle-class, and not representative of the local population. Student contact with black patients was therefore relatively infrequent, as was the discussion of ethnic and racial diversity in their training programme, except for one of their assessment criteria described as 'awareness of patient's cultural needs'. Thus once again students were expected to meet patients' so-called cultural needs without discussing what this meant or being adequately prepared to do so. Current thinking amongst educators for a multi-racial Britain, for example, was critical of subsuming race and ethnicity under the relatively innocuous term 'culture'[7]. During their ward experiences, therefore, students were exposed to racial stereotyping without being offered any alternative perspectives with which to challenge them.

Take Miss Baxter, suffering from Parkinson's disease, who was a large black woman in her sixties and described predictably by the ward staff as a 'big black mama'. Miss Baxter, like many patients of her age and condition, snored loudly at night, and many of her neighbouring patients described her amongst themselves as an 'animal'. The staff and students were aware of the offensive way in which Miss Baxter was referred to, but did not articulate it as a racist stereotype (as clearly it was), nor do anything to dispel it amongst the patients.

Once Miss Baxter's behaviour won the nurses' approval, she acquired another set of stereotypes during the ward handovers where she was described as 'ever such a nice lady' and 'very pleasant and smiling'. Weren't 'big black mamas' supposed to be smiling? Thus any racial stereotyping by either nurses or patients was left unchallenged and without appropriate consciousness raising, to be reproduced, potentially, at a later date by students.

In this chapter I have described how nurses define the physical, technical and emotional components of their work according to medical specialties. But students frequently found themselves in emotionally charged situations. These situations went beyond the medical and technical definitions of their training and back to nursing as people work. This was reflected in the way in which students used patients' personal characteristics as well as what was 'wrong' with them as a way of describing their work and learning. Thus patients' age, gender, racial characteristics and whether they were appreciative also shaped the way in which they saw their work.

Violent incidents are used to articulate the gendered nature of the social relations between patients and nurses and the high expectations to maintain an outward appearance of calm, even when feeling physically and sexually threatened.

Students frequently engaged in emotional labour in these emotionally charged situations. Often they experienced anxiety and stress because their emotional labour was neither formally recognised nor valued as part of 'real' nursing (with the possible exceptions of oncology and psychiatry) nor incorporated into the theoretical and practical organisation of their training. How then did emotional labour, the invisible and undervalued component of nursing get reproduced in the wards?

5 The ward sister and the infrastructure of emotion work: making it visible on the ward

In the 'real world' of the ward, emotion work was neither formally recognised nor valued as part of nursing. But nurses still engaged in it. What, then, were the conditions that permitted its production and reproduction? My research suggests that the answer lies with the ward sister, who, as the architect of nursing work and organisation, sets the emotional agenda (i.e. the feeling rules) of the ward. When the nurses felt appreciated and supported emotionally by the ward sisters, they not only had a role model for emotionally explicit patient care, but they also felt able to care for patients in this way.

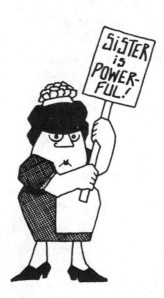

(Source: Cath Jackson)

In Chapter 2 we met the ward sister who was the City 'type', everyone's ideal who was calm, kind and considerate, but also got the work done on time. This description contrasted strongly with the traditional image of the ward sister as a battleaxe or dragon whose authoritarian behaviour made students and patients fear and avoid her. A patient who had been in and out of hospital over the last 20 years thought that ward sisters had changed from her first days as a patient. She said: 'Ward sisters are mostly nice these days; perhaps they've softened. They get to know people more, rather than being superior as in the past'.

Questionnaire data presented in the previous chapter, however, show that 'hierarchical and unfriendly staff relations' were still a major source of anxiety and stress for students because of the feelings they generated.

The City nurse was 'attractive', almost like a model (perfection), unlike the traditional ward sister portrayed as 'frumpy' and 'middle-aged'. But they were similar in that they both always got the work done on time, i.e. they were competent and efficient.

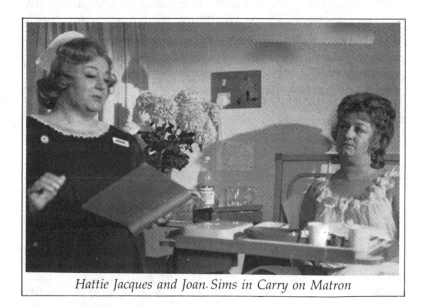

Hattie Jacques and Joan Sims in Carry on Matron

Emergencies and emotions

Take the following incident, which took place during participant observation. It's a Thursday morning. Things are quite slow on Kinder ward today: no doctors' rounds, no new patients for admission, everyone except Bobbi in Bed 4 able to get up and about. We're making the beds and feeling quite relaxed, chatting to each other and the patients. Sister is busy on the telephone. Suddenly there's an urgent shout from the bathroom. It's staff nurse Sue: 'Robin!' she shouts. Everyone knows immediately what's up. It's Robin, and he's stopped breathing again. This has been happening with increasing regularity since Robin, aged 19, was admitted with a drug overdose some days ago. We're not sure what the trigger is, but it's very unpredictable and very frightening. Maybe he's still managing to get his friends to bring drugs into the hospital for him. But whatever the cause we've got to get him breathing again, and fast. An emergency call is put through to the hospital resuscitation team, but what counts most is the immediate action we can take on the ward.

We're a pretty inexperienced team this morning. Two of the students have never seen a respiratory arrest (the technical term for when someone stops breathing) and Sue sounds really desperate, because although she's a staff nurse, she hasn't either. I have to dig in to my memory to remember the routine, but, as sister says later, she's seen more emergencies than had hot dinners. And it shows. She's there in a second, telling Sue and one of the students to move Robin from the cramped bathroom to the open space of the ward. She's already grabbed the emergency box, and has the airway inserted and the ambubag attached to inflate Robin's lungs whilst calling out instructions to fetch emergency oxygen, the suction machine and intravenous equipment. She never raises her voice, but speaks calmly and clearly whilst working deftly with the ambubag, and now the suction catheter, to get Robin breathing again. She congratulates Ellie, the first-year student, for remembering to bring the correct size of catheter.

By now, the emergency team has arrived, and I receive my orders to draw up the drugs to correct Robin's electrolytes. I can't believe how much my hands are shaking, and my mouth feels very dry! I cast a quick glance around me. The ward looks like a war zone. Robin now lies prone on a bed, surrounded by tubes and people, blood oozing from a head graze, sister and a couple of doctors beside him. The students respond efficiently to their instructions, but their ashen faces are a sure sign that they're feeling the strain. I know I am. But we work hard at controlling our panic and we're inspired by sister, who carries on calmly telling us what to do. Then there are the other patients looking on, horror-struck. There isn't much you can do to protect them in an open ward like this, but a visiting social worker leads those who are able, Pied Piper-like, to the relative quiet of the day room.

Robin is now breathing spontaneously and the immediate danger has passed. He begins to regain consciousness. Sister decides she wants some time alone with him, and draws the curtains round his bed. Everyone begins to leave, removing their equipment and debris with them. Sister fetches a bowl of water and towels and gently washes Robin, trying at the same time to find out what's going on psychologically for him. She's with him for nearly an hour.

Meanwhile, the life of the ward slowly returns to normal and as the next shift has already arrived, Sue sends the morning students off to lunch. When they return, sister is ready for them. Having left Robin sleeping, she now takes the students to the day room and asks them how they are feeling after the morning's emergency. They talk about the strains of having Robin as a patient, but also they are congratulated for their prompt action. Everyone leaves the room looking visibly brighter with smiles on their faces and ready to meet the next emergency in the knowledge of a job well done. And Robin, as I'm told later by Ellie, has the students on his side. They don't see him as a deviant, taking up valuable resources, but as one of society's casualties to be supported and helped.

Next day, Robin is well enough to walk to the flower shop and buy sister some roses with promises that he'll let the doctors refer him to a drug treatment centre. Only time will tell if he'll get there, but at the moment he's quiet and the tension on the ward generated by his emotional and physical instability temporarily decreases. The students feel secure that sister takes the emergencies 'in her stride', 'no-one panics' and, as a first-year student points out, 'the trained staff asked me if I felt all right when it was all over'.

On another ward, a third-year student fares less well during an emergency as a consequence of a ward sister who she perceives as authoritarian and traditional, and lacking in either calmness or consideration for her juniors. The student is involved in caring for an unconscious patient whose condition suddenly deteriorates. She calls the sister, who comes quickly to the patient's bedside followed closely by two doctors. The student is told immediately to suction the secretions from the patient's airway. The sister's tone is cold and mechanical. The student quickly dons gloves, assembles the suction equipment and turns on the suction machine. She then moves purposefully towards the patient and begins to insert the suction catheter into his mouth to take away any secretions which may have caused him to choke. In her haste to obey the sister's instructions, she forgets the golden rule 'before any procedure always tell the patient, even when unconscious, what you are going to do'. Her omission immediately provokes the sister to snap at her for failing to warn the patient that he was about to be subject to an invasive procedure.

The student is so shocked and upset at being spoken to in this way that before she knows what is happening the tears are streaming down her cheeks. She swallows hard to conceal any sounds and hopes that the sister will not notice as she recovers herself sufficiently to carry on with the suctioning procedure. The sister and doctors nudge each other and exchange meaningful glances about the student's tears, but do not say anything to her, either in comfort or reprimand. She leaves the patient's bedside at the first possible opportunity and goes straight to the bathroom where she immediately bursts into the sobs she has suppressed in public.

Later, she told me the reasons for her reactions. Firstly, she had felt tense and anxious at the patient's sudden deterioration. Secondly, suctioning patients to clear their airway was still a relatively unfamiliar and frightening procedure to her, so that she had been concentrating hard on the technical task in hand. When the sister abruptly broke into her concentration, she was genuinely startled, then shocked and humiliated that she had overlooked such a basic principle as to warn the patient of the impending procedure. She felt even more humiliated when the sister and doctors, rather than being sympathetic, reacted in a dumb show behind her back. She felt that the sister had made her look stupid in front of the doctors and had undermined her confidence.

These two accounts illustrate some of the stresses and tensions surrounding the emergency care of acutely ill patients. They also demonstrate the effects of the sister's management style on the emotional well-being of patients and nurses.

In the first account, the sister demonstrated calmness, competency, kindness and understanding, which not only assisted the students to manage Robin's respiratory arrest technically but to support him emotionally. If, for example, she had left him to recover on his own instead of spending time talking to him, she might have indicated to the students that Robin was a lost cause, not worth the effort because he was not trying to help himself get over his drug problem. Instead, she showed that she cared for his psychological as well as physical well-being and averted the situation in another ward where a student told me that the nursing staff believed that 'patients with drug problems are just a waste of time. They're a working class problem and why should they be treated?'. The sister on Kinder ward avoided labelling Robin as a 'problem' patient and helped the students to invest in him emotionally rather than forcing them to withdraw, like Tracy in the last chapter because of lack of support, or the students in Chapter 3 who took their cues from trained staff and avoided certain patients.

In the second account, the ward sister responded quickly and competently to an emergency. She might even have been seen to have the patient's psychological well-being at heart in that she reminded the student to tell the patient what she was doing. But the abrupt and impersonal way in which she handled the student's omission, and seemingly colluded with the doctors, made the student feel humiliated and unsupported. Under such conditions, the student temporarily lost both her technical and emotional confidence to care for patients.

The sisters in both accounts are judged on their speed, technical competency and their interpersonal skills. The first sister like the City Hospital nurse, is 'everybody's ideal'; a sort of 'super-nurse'. One student, a first-year, told me how much she admired her because:

She was always there when it counted. She'd always give us support. She really didn't make you feel stupid and the way she reacted in an emergency [said admiringly] ....

The second sister, although technically competent and efficient, fails in the student's eyes because she did not support her, and worse, made her feel stupid.

Let's look more closely at the characteristics of 'everybody's ideal' ward sister and nurse first described in Chapter 1.

Everybody's ideal: characteristics of ward sisters and nurses

What begins to emerge is that even though students admired technical competency and specialist (medical) knowledge in their ward sister they also saw her as the key person in setting the emotional climate of the ward. An emotionally caring climate made the student feel cared for and thus better able to care for others.

We saw in Chapter 2 that the ideal nurse, the 'City type' was modelled on a ward sister. As I talked more to both trained and student nurses about their idea of a 'good' nurse it became clear that the 'ideal' characteristics of both nurse and ward sister were virtually interchangeable.

Thus, the 'ideal' nurse, frequently modelled on a much admired ward sister, represents the high expectations that nurses have for themselves and each other, which are passed on from one generation to the next. Technical competency and specialist knowledge no longer dominate the picture, and the importance of the emotional component of caring as an explicit management style begins to emerge. The following quotations demonstrate the constancy of the characteristics of the 'ideal' nurse, passed on from one generation of nurses to the next and their admiration of and aspiration to both technical competency and emotional literacy. Ward sisters with at least 20 years' nursing experience had the following to say about nurses they identified from their past as their own ideal.

For one sister, her role model was 'a very good organiser, a very good practical nurse and she really cared for the well-being of the patients. She really cared for them as a person'.

Another ward sister still felt daunted (like the student who described the ward sister who was the City type and everybody's ideal) by the person who had taught her 'a lot. She never seemed to make mistakes. Every thing she did was perfect [like the City sister who was just like a 'model']. Her management. Everything. She's the sort of person I really couldn't fault'.

74

The sister summed up her ideal nurse as 'competent and caring. She had very good practical skills, but she would do the little things for patients and leave them feeling very much better'.

Another ward sister spoke about two sisters whom she had admired for their hard work, high standards and personal involvement with staff and patients. These personal qualities were the antithesis of the traditional ward sister described above, who provoked fear and anxiety and made junior nurses feel stupid. She said:

> I think involvement is so important rather than this hierarchy system where the sister made people so nervous that you were actually afraid to express how you felt about anything and you couldn't develop your own role because you were suppressed by her system.

All these sisters agreed that organisation, technical competency and high standards were important elements in a ward manager, but most importantly this was incomplete without a 'caring side' which let their juniors express how they felt and left the patients feeling better (i.e. this caring side was about how people *felt*).

Students who had been training as nurses from between a few weeks and three years identified similar qualities in their ward sisters. But there was one characteristic which the sisters didn't mention that the students identified as being particularly important for them as trainees. They liked to know what was expected of them at the beginning of a ward allocation. One student said:

> Sister on this specialist surgical ward was very good. She sat me down on my first shift and said 'This is what I expect from a third year', so I knew where I stood from the beginning. I said to her 'If every sister did that, the wards would run so much smoother'.

Another student expressed a similar view about a sister on a medical ward:

> I think the whole ward was run very smoothly because you knew where you were. She had rules. She let you know what the rules were.

The students also liked to know that the rules and expectations on a ward were consistent and that they would not be 'worrying about someone coming round your neck saying "don't do that, do this"'. Consistency of rules and expectations on the part of the sister was one of the ways in which she created a supportive and relaxed ward atmosphere. One of the oncology ward sisters was frequently described in this way. A third-year student told me that 'it was very easy to feel at ease on this ward' which she thought was 'very good for nursing care, if you feel relaxed with *people*'. A first-year student described in more detail how the sister made people 'feel at ease' and 'relaxed'. 'We had a very easy-going relationship. Everybody was called by their first names and you had a real laugh'.

But the student was very quick to point out that the standard of nursing did not drop because of the 'easy-going relationship'; rather it helped to make the care of very sick patients 'top priority'.

Another student, previously quoted in Chapter 1, explained that:

When I know that the ward sister cares then I feel a bit more at ease. Otherwise I feel that I have to take the whole caring attitude of the whole ward on my shoulders.

If that caring atmosphere or attitude did not exist, then the student, a third-year, felt responsible for creating it herself.

Coming through from these accounts was the connection between the creation of a 'caring' atmosphere (feeling relaxed with people; easy-going relationship between sister and staff; having a laugh; being on first name terms; not having to take responsibility for the caring attitude of the whole ward) and feeling better able to care for patients.

Students also admired ward sisters who took their time to talk to patients and their relatives, staying over time to do this 'if someone is upset'. This behaviour signified to students that 'sister is genuinely concerned about the patients'.

As one student said 'you picked this concern up so that everything people wanted was done. I mean it wasn't done grudgingly, it was done well. I would really want to do things for people on that ward'.

But it was not only on a ward where emotional labour was legitimised (i.e. oncology) that students described their ideal sisters. A surgical ward sister for example was described as 'very competent, very nice, very funny. She makes the ward happy'.

The sister's ability to create good social relations among nursing staff was a critical component of the ward atmosphere as the following quotations illustrate.

> Sisters are critical because of their influence on staff nurses. They in turn influence how the students work and on the way they feel, their morale.

> Sister's attitude is very important. On sister depends the happiness of staff nurses and students.

The significance of creating good social relations between the nurses on the ward becomes evident when we consider the hierarchical nature of nursing. We can draw on the example given by the ward sister above to illustrate the potential use of this 'hierarchy system' to make subordinates feel nervous, afraid, suppressed. A student gives similar insights:

> Sister is undoubtedly critical. Sister is undoubtedly the key. I believe in the fact that it all goes up in the system and I feel the sister of the ward she sets the pace. She informs the staff nurses and they will do things according to her wishes, even if [as happens on some wards] they totally disagree with things she has given them to do.

A student who had just finished on a ward described the effects of an authoritarian management style which produced anxiety in the staff nurses 'because they felt responsible to sister'. In turn the staff nurses felt they had to 'check' the students 'every inch of the way and they were on your back and badgering you and hassling you all the time'.

Students were also very critical of ward sisters, and sometimes their staff nurses, who sat in their offices behind closed doors 'sending the orders down'. The physical separation of the trained staff from the students reinforced the hierarchical nature of the social relations between them, and as one student observed:

> Any socialising that goes on is between students. The trained staff never really get to know us as people. On the last ward

you weren't allowed in the office if anybody trained was there. We'd have to go in the day room with the patients.

The mark of the good ward sister was the one who was out there on the ward caring for patients alongside students. Through her contact with patients she 'kept in touch' and was able 'to see the amount of work students do'. As another student said 'When they're out there on the ward you feel you can go and talk to them. They're much more approachable than when they're sitting in their little office'.

The ideal sister did not supervise in the way of the sister who created anxiety for her staff and students by checking 'every inch of the way'. Rather she took an 'interest in what you are doing and how you are *feeling* about the ward. She makes sure the work is allocated fairly and within the students' capabilities. She also says "I'll come and help you" if you haven't done it before'.

A tutor summed up the characteristics of the 'ideal ward environment' created by the sister which confirmed the students' views described above. She said:

The ideal environment is where there is consistency, teamwork and where you don't have a hierarchical 'us and them' situation. The students see fairness and consistency because the sister and staff nurses roll up their sleeves and work.

Another tutor described similar characteristics based on two actual (surgical) ward sisters working at City at that time.

These two sisters create an efficient and effective environment and they are regarded with affection by the nurses. The atmosphere on their wards is very safe. They are extremely approachable and very clear-cut in what they want and the students know exactly where they are with them.

I was interested by her description, because the language she used was reminiscent of that used to define emotional labour in the sense of producing in others a sense of being cared for (the sisters were extremely approachable and clear-cut, i.e. consistent) in a convivial (the sisters were regarded with affection) *safe place* (the wards had a 'very safe atmosphere').

Further evidence that students felt more able to care for patients if the trained staff were working alongside them and taking an interest in them is summed up by a student at the end of her training. She said: 'I think students work jolly hard if they are working with somebody who understands them a bit more and thanks them at the end of the shift, rather than bossing them around all the time'.

The indicators of 'caring' management styles, described above, might be interpreted as the sister's recognition of the importance of the emotional components of nursing to the care of both students and patients. In order to care for the emotional needs of patients and nurses, sisters created feeling rules that valued personhood, good social relations and emotions as part of the work. They put themselves in direct patient contact alongside the students rather than keeping their distance by staying in their offices and 'sending the orders down'.

The hierarchical ward sister also created feeling rules based on hierarchy, authority and often high standards of patient care that were unattainable even by them. These sisters were often perfectionists and prioritised technical competency and efficiency at the expense of their own, their juniors' and patients' emotional needs. Students and staff nurses on these wards were likely to experience negative feelings (fear, anxiety, suppression) as a consequence of the sister's hierarchical management style. One staff nurse told me, for example, how one of the ward sisters had such high standards that she couldn't take working with her anymore. She said: 'Sister would pick up something [e.g. a mistake] and you'd think, "Why didn't I think of that?!"'.

Students described feelings in their written questionnaire comments that were triggered by hierarchical management styles:

Confidence undermined, so that it was difficult to show initiative; made to feel inadequate if uncertain about care; on the defensive because of criticism.

As one student commented about the ward sister above: because you were just never able to reach her high standards she rarely gave positive encouragement – only negative reactions and reports.

One student concluded: 'Fear isn't a good way to learn to care. Mutual respect is the best. If you feel appreciated you try

79

to live up to the faith people have in you. It's a very strong stimulus'.

The relationship between caring for nurses and caring for patients was articulated by both students and patients. Two third-year students expressed the view, for example, that patients like nurses were sensitive to ward atmospheres created by the sister (cf. Revans, 1964). Patients knew if the students were not happy or morale was low. In one student's experience, this had resulted in patients not wanting to bother the 'poor nurses'.

Another student described how patients responded to the ward atmosphere. She said:

I think that most of the patients are quite happy with their care on most of the wards. Well practically everything is done for them. But that doesn't mean that patients aren't aware if there is a tense atmosphere on some wards. They can sort of sense the stress. It filters down to them and it makes them unhappy, whereas on other wards they're much more relaxed.

A patient also told me: 'If staff work well with sister then the atmosphere of the ward is well. They shouldn't be frightened of her'.

In summary, these accounts suggest that nurses were looking for supportive sisters who gave them back their personhood, which the hierarchy threatened to take away. Sisters who related to students hierarchically made them feel frightened, anxious and defensive. When the nurses felt appreciated and supported emotionally by the sisters, they not only had a role model for emotionally explicit patient care but they also felt better able to care for patients in this way. Patients and nurses were sensitive to the ward atmosphere and social relations created by the sister. The assumption is that technical and physical labour are enhanced when underpinned by an emotionally explicit caring style.

Producing and reproducing emotional labour in the ward

So in what ways did the sisters manage their wards to set the emotional tone to make the students, and hence the patients, feel safe and cared for in a convivial environment as opposed to frightened, anxious and defensive? How were the feeling rules of the ward made explicit?

The majority of ward sisters had chosen to work on specific wards because of their interest in a particular specialty. Most of them had been students at City Hospital or another teaching hospital first before taking specialist training of their choice. Post-registration courses in critical care nursing were particularly popular for prospective sisters wanting to take charge of general medical and surgical wards. Courses were also available to those with a specialist interest in neurology, oncology, cardiology and orthopaedics.

The staff nurses had usually worked on the ward as students and had decided both that they liked the specialty and the sister's particular style.

One sister explained how she recruited her staff nurses. She said:

> I suppose they recruit themselves really. They work on the wards as students, the majority of them, and then if they enjoyed the ward they ask if they can come back for consolidation and if there's a vacancy and if they're interested and they're satisfactory at interview, they're appointed.

But the implication of what the sister is saying is that she recruited staff nurses who would reproduce an explicitly emotional caring style.

A staff nurse explained how another sister's management style which she described as 'laid-back' (i.e. calm and easygoing) had been a reason to apply to work on a particular ward. She said: 'Patients like it; staff like it, and she's one of the few sisters who actually nurses patients'. The importance of the sister being out there on the ward giving patient care was once more in evidence, as well as the effects of a particular management style on both patients and nurses.

Thus, the sisters and staff nurses not only chose to work together because they liked each other's philosophy and style, but developed into a cohesive group over a period of at least a year. Students and patients, on the other hand, stayed for much shorter periods on the wards and did not usually have much say over their placements or admissions. Students stayed on the ward for an eight-week period, whereas the average length of stay for most patients in the City Hospital at the time of the

81

study was less than a week. Each group was there with its different perspectives: the students to learn; the patients to face illness and treatment in order, they hoped, to recover; and the sisters and staff nurses to organise their care. This also entailed managing doctors' treatment orders and regimes as part of the competing nurturing/responsibilty, technical–economic and scientific rationalities[1].

The accounts at the beginning of this chapter show us that the sister was crucial in setting the emotional tone or feeling rules of the ward, and it is likely that her work preferences and priorities were determined by her own particular rationality of care rather than the medical speciality of the ward. Furthermore, the person-orientated approach of the nursing process was more in keeping with a nurturing rationality.

Like the teachers, many of the ward sisters had trained in the pre-nursing process days, when a biomedical approach to nursing based on scientific rationality was taken for granted. Task-orientated care designed to get the work done and minimise close interpersonal nurse–patient encounters was the order of the day[2].

Other factors also shape hospital routines and work organisation. When sisters are charged with the care of, say, 20 patients and 15 nurses, two-thirds of whom are untrained, the origins of task-orientated nursing become evident. Many sisters find it easier to supervise and control the students, who are at the front line of care, by adherence to tasks and routines rather than giving them responsibility for planning their own patient-centred care (Davies, 1976; Proctor, 1989).

I can remember, as a student, receiving my orders in the morning to do all the temperatures for patients or make the beds, or bathe all those requiring bedbaths. Then every few hours, I would go round to all the patients confined to bed and give them a bedpan and later a back-rub. Each nurse was allocated her task according to her seniority. In all, a patient could be nursed by four or five different nurses in a day, with none of them being personally responsible for their whole care. The ward sister and her deputies, the staff nurses, allocated the tasks but, as Bendall (1975) showed, they did not always find out to what extent their orders had been carried out. Take for instance the patient who was supposed to be confined to a chair by her bed and who spent 43 minutes sitting in the toilet, taken there and then forgotten by a passing nurse. No written or verbal report of the incident was ever recorded. Bendall saw the incident and its invisibility as a consequence of nurses being responsible for carrying out a number of tasks for 20 or more patients rather than being responsible for the whole care of any one patient.

Such an extreme incident of the type described by Bendall was unlikely to occur at the City Hospital. For one thing, the patients had an electrical call system which they were always instructed to use before being left for any length of time either behind curtains or in the bathroom. Nurses usually responded fairly quickly to the call system, and the longest I saw a patient being kept waiting was about nine minutes on a busy evening shift. Furthermore, as we discussed in Chapter 3, nurses had some sense of the nursing process as a patient- rather than task-orientated work method. Although on all the wards I worked one or two nurses were assigned on each shift to look after a group of patients (average of six per shift) some sisters still operated a routine which required that students performed certain tasks by certain times. I have been called in by a student to finish bathing a patient so that she could go and take her coffee break before the prescribed time. Many's the time it's been, 'Have you finished your patients Pam? Could you finish off Mrs Graham for me?' Usually Mrs Graham knew me because I might have looked after her on previous occasions, but I wasn't necessarily up to date with her current care and it seemed absurd for one person to begin her bath and another to complete it. But the student was concerned to get all the baths done in time, so although the sister might allocate the work by patients she still made it clear that there were certain routine tasks on each shift that had to be completed.

But the extreme routines of the past had virtually disappeared from City. Take the example of the 'back trolley'. On one ward, the sister, staff nurses and I were discussing 'the old days', when every four hours nurses had progressed along the ward with their back trolley, applying massage and a variety of concoctions (alcohol, talcum powder, soap and water) to the pressure areas of bedridden patients. The routine, known as 'the back round' was thought to prevent pressure sores. Some years ago, the use of the back trolley and pressure area routines was condemned as doing more harm than good, because not only did they damage the skin, but they diverted attention from removing the main cause of sores i.e. pressure (Norton, 1962).

The staff nurses who had trained at City and had been qualified for about a year were fascinated by the discussion because they had never heard of 'a back trolley', but more to the point found the idea of being allocated tasks (such as a back round) rather than patients for a shift totally unfamiliar to their way of working at City.

Yet many patient-centred tasks and routines persisted on the wards, shaped by medical diagnosis and treatment (doctors' rounds and varieties of diagnostic tests and therapies on and off the ward) as part of the 'assembly line care of the sick' motivated by scientific rationality[3]. On some wards, sisters as well as doctors were motivated by a scientific rather than a nurturing rationality which led them to organise the nursing work in this way.

On a cardiology ward, for example, the sister placed great emphasis on maintaining accurate fluid balance charts. This activity was important for monitoring a patient's cardiac function. However, one first-ward student became so anxious about filling in her fluid balance charts that she concentrated on the task rather than the characteristics of the individual patient. One of her allocated patients was to go to the operating theatre. An NBM (nil by mouth) sign had been attached to the bed. The student went through all her patients' charts (which included the lady about to go to theatre) assuming that because the after-lunch drink had just been served, rather than disturb the patients, all she needed to do was fill in the standard amount of fluid equivalent to a cup against the appropriate time. All hell was let loose when a staff nurse discovered that the fasting patient had supposedly had a cup of tea. The student was sent for and an explanation demanded. How come this patient about to go to theatre had received a cup of tea? It soon became clear that the student had based her entry on routine because of her lack of experience and anxiety to get through tasks. She told me later that she could not believe how 'stupid' she had been. But she had also been made to feel stupid by the trained staff. 'I knew Dorothy was going for an op.', she said, 'I knew she was "nil by mouth", I knew she wasn't taking food but I wasn't sure whether that meant drinks as well and I was so worried about getting my fluid charts done'.

A third-year student was critical of the emphasis on routines on this and other wards, believing that it prevented students from questioning their care. She said: 'On some wards the care is just too routinised. You just do things and you don't question'. The incident of the inexperienced student and the fluid balance chart certainly suggested this to be the case.

The technical–economic rationality is no more evident than in the domestic organisation of a 500 bed hospital. Meals and ward cleaning, for example, are organised around a predetermined time allowance or timetable based on a male concept of time[4].

A student only weeks into her training, motivated to care for people rather than diseases, soon realised that the running of a hospital was in opposition to the people-centred ethos of the nursing process and hence a nurturing rationality. She said:

I mean hospitals aren't run for the individual patient, they're run for everybody, aren't they? It would be nice if they could be geared to each person but they can't really, can they?

Her question is a pertinent one and has been at the centre of a number of research studies. How possible is it to meet individual needs within an institution? King and colleagues (1971) used Goffman's typology of total institutions (1968) for measuring the degree of client-centredness within childcare institutions. Miller and Gwynne (1972) discovered that chronically disabled residents in long-stay institutions were either encouraged as individuals (the horticultural model of care) or were the recipients of impersonal routines (the warehousing model of care). Evers (1984) applied their analysis to the care of the elderly in the wards of a geriatric hospital. She found that the different orientations on a ward towards either the horticultural or the warehousing model was primarily dependent on the ward sister[5]. Fretwell (1982) also found that sisters in general wards made their own choices about their work preferences and priorities[6].

I was particularly interested in these findings, because they showed that client or institutional orientation on a ward or unit depended on the attitudes of the supervisor or sister. Similar findings emerged from my own study, focusing particularly on how the sister set the emotional tone of the ward. It was this emotional tone and how she set it (her emotional management style) that in part answered the student's question as to how possible it was to gear the needs of the institution to 'each person'. I found that when a ward sister had an express commitment to the nursing process person-centered philosophy she was more likely to use it as a work method to create the infrastructure which allowed the production and reproduction of emotional labour in her ward. How did she do this?

Reproducing emotional labour, management styles and the nursing process

The sisters on the wards I observed were all committed to the person-orientated approach of the nursing process, but they interpreted its work method in different ways. They were all patient-centred to varying degrees, but the amount of contact they had with doctors varied according to specialty. In the more specialised wards, where patients were undergoing a battery of medical tests and investigations, the sisters and doctors worked more closely together. On the general medical wards, more patients were well advanced in their illness trajectory. Often they were entering a chronic phase and tended to be more dependent on nursing care than medical intervention. Here, the sisters and doctors had less contact with each other. Whatever the case, the sisters did not lose sight of either the patients or the students, but some clearly saw patient care as their top priority whilst others saw teaching students as an integral part of that priority. The sister on Edale ward, for example, said: 'I see that it's my responsiblity to ensure the patients get good care and one of the ways to ensure this is to teach the students how'. The students recognised the sister's commitment to teaching and gave Edale top ratings on the learning environment questionnaires (see Tables E8, E9 and E10 in Appendix E).

Emotion work was not officially legitimised by the medical specialty on these four wards. Even though a number of patients on all the wards were suffering from cancer, because none of them were officially oncology wards, death and dying were not on the medically legitimised agenda.

On Ronda ward, many of the patients were suffering from a variety of chronic illnesses, ranging from respiratory to Alzheimer's disease, and although many of the patients were elderly the physicians still worked in an interventionist and curative way.

But the sister was more orientated towards emotion work compared with many of her colleagues. One student told me how unusual she thought this was on a general ward, adding

86

that she thought that Sister Ronda worked more in the style of an oncology ward sister.

Another student told me how she had gone 'overboard' for Ronda ward and its elderly patient population:

My set [classmates] thought I was mad because the ward has this reputation of being just basic nursing. But Sister Ronda made me realise what an art it is to care for people who can't do very much for themselves and who rely on good personal relationships.

Yet another student, quoted in Chapter 4, who described the mechanisms used on a psychiatric ward to focus on the emotional aspects of work, told me that very few general ward sisters worked in this way. She mentioned two sisters, one of whom was Sister Ronda, the other a ward sister on a care of the elderly ward who did. When I asked her why she thought they were able to work in this way, she said:

They are both open to change. On most general wards you are expected to support a patient in depression but you're not supported yourself. You are expected to treat the patients psychologically, but nobody tells you how to do that. But these two sisters do. They are very open to change with regard to the nursing process and they try desperately hard each shift to do what is right.

The implication of this last statement was that the ward sister assessed both student and patient need on every shift. During participant observation I observed Sister Ronda doing this. She wanted to know how people were feeling in order to suggest ways of caring for psychological as well as technical and physical needs (cf. below the ward where psychosocial care was all part of the 'scientific approach').

On first meeting Sister Ronda, I was immediately struck by the warm and open way she related to people. She was very welcoming to me, even though I was a total stranger until then. She quickly established a rapport with her clear gaze, responsive facial expressions and a reassuring hand on my forearm. During the subsequent weeks of fieldwork, I noticed that Sister Ronda spent considerable proportions of her time talking to patients, a characteristic which provoked one student to describe her as 'being very into her patients'. During my research, Sister Ronda was the only person who clearly articulated the importance of patients' emotional support to nurses, especially those who were regularly admitted to her ward over the years. She valued their friendships and felt that nurses were able to learn so much from them as they faced their chronic illnesses with courage and determination. I remember being momentarily taken by surprise when one of Ronda ward's regular patients was re-admitted. She and the sister greeted each other warmly, each giving the other a hug. I reflected on the incident for some time and then began to understand why it had made an impression on me. It was because I still expected nurses, especially ward sisters, to be distant and cool from their patients, applying their 'no touch' aseptic surgical techniques to their personal relationships.

But this was not Sister Ronda's way. She was clearly motivated by a nurturing rationality that put people at the centre of care rather than sticking to rigid timetables and routines. As one student put it: 'Sister Ronda doesn't mind how long it takes, but other sisters want you to get on with their routines'.

Another student described the sister's emphasis on communication rather than tasks: 'Sister is atypical. She emphasises communication. She doesn't mind if you sit and talk to patients and don't get the bedbaths done'.

Comparing another ward, where a scientific rather than a nurturing rationality motivated the trained staff, she continued: 'The staff are not madly geared to that sort of thing [communication]. They run the ward on a scientific approach, which means that psychosocial care is included as part of that. It isn't given any special priority or anything'.

The consequences of being encouraged to be 'psychosocially orientated' and to talk with patients as part of the work is expressed by a student in the following way: 'Sister is very psychosocially based, you feel bad if you can't talk to the patients as the sister expects it'.

The following comment represented a recurrent theme amongst staff and students on Ronda ward: 'You nearly always go off duty feeling you've not done everything. You often wonder whether it really is because of the amount of work or the way you organise it'.

One reason why the nurses never felt that they had finished their work at the end of the shift was because they experienced

Sister Ronda's emphasis on communication as extra to an extremely physically demanding workload.

The 'laid back' management style of Sister Windermere's ward was described by one student as preferable to Sister Ronda's approach because it meant that the ward was run so well that it *left time* (my emphasis) for students to use their initiatives to do extras for the patients 'like talking to them'. There was enough evidence however, that students didn't start out feeling that talking to patients was an 'extra'. One student on her first ward, which was not Sister Ronda's, experienced the pressure of always being seen to be 'doing things' other than talking. She said:

I do love it when you have time for the patients. I really enjoy it. I get frustrated when there isn't time, time to sit and chat. I do like sitting there, but the trained staff always make me feel as if I should be doing other things.

Patients, as well as students, often marginalised 'talking' with nurses as an extra. I experienced this early on in the fieldwork when I was sitting talking to a patient about her illness and treatment. At one point in the discussion she suddenly interjected: 'Oh I'm sorry I'd better not keep you from your work'. When I explained that our discussion was part of my work, she relaxed and carried on talking.

However, the situation also occurred where the physical labour could be so demanding that emotional labour took second priority. One patient told me, for example, how when the staffing levels were low, nurses would be so rushed that even though they began conversations they might be called away before they had time to finish them.

These descriptions of time and the workload have resonances with the notion of work being constrained by a predetermined time allowance or timetable associated with a male concept of time. Students found themselves caught between the competing rationalities, not only of hospital administrators and doctors, but also their ward sisters. In the mid-1980s, Sister Ronda's obvious concern for people and recognition of communication and the development of good personal relations as part of the work was seen by many students as 'atypical' but also mildly eccentric and at times impractical. Furthermore, her emphasis on people rather than tasks could be seen as changing a system that served as a defence against student anxiety[7].

The association between a people-orientated approach to nursing and the practice of the nursing process was personified in Sister Ronda. She had the reputation throughout the hospital of being one of the sisters who was most committed to the nursing process. To the students this meant that she put patients at the centre of care, carefully identifying their needs and planning their nursing with the students. She approached patient care from a nursing rather than a biomedical approach, encouraging students to identify patients' needs based on Roper's activities of living (Roper, 1976). Personal relationships were at the centre of her interactions both with patients and students and emotional needs were openly identified and articulated. The students' top questionnaire ratings of the positive staff relations on Ronda ward were evidence of this (Table E11 in Appendix E).

In what ways then did Sister Ronda organise and manage nursing in a way that made her management style emotionally different to many of her colleagues?

First of all, it was the way in which she allocated and distributed the work based on individual nurses caring for specific patients. Many of the students, used to the more usual practice on other wards of patient-centred tasks found Sister Ronda's emphasis on patient-centred care difficult to deal with. Their reaction was part of feeling that organising care in a patient-centred way took more time than was available, because it also meant 'getting to know them' especially for patients who had a high level of physical dependency. Getting to know patients and being in continuous contact with them also meant that nurses were required to manage their feelings more than when they operated at the level of getting through tasks. As one student allocated to Ronda ward put it:

I was looking after these four highly dependent patients. And it was a struggle to get through the work. When I was giving Mrs Clark a bed bath I was interrupted seven times to get commodes and things for the other patients. At one point I got so frustrated I kicked a stool in between Mrs Clark and Marion's bed. Marion noticed and called me over. She was quite upset because she thought I was angry with her. I felt so ashamed but I also thought to myself, this is what happens when patient allocation goes too far.

The conflict between getting through the work and relating on a one-to-one basis with patients was no more evident than in the student's failure to suppress feelings of frustration, followed by shame when one patient misinterpreted her behaviour.

Another student, speaking for many, was reluctant to look after patients on a continuous basis during their hospital stay. One reason for her reluctance seemed to be associated with the increased demand for emotional labour. She said:

It depends really on striking the balance between getting to know the patients well and knowing what's going on in the rest of the ward. And not letting say a certain patient getting to the point of irritating you. Because it does happen if you're working for days and days and days looking after the same person who is aggressive or rude. By the end of it your patience just wears thin.

On the majority of the wards the trained staff held the view that students should be given some choice over who they looked after and for how long. As one student explained (and which I saw verified time and time again during the report), the trained staff would say:

Who looked after so and so today? And they would then let another nurse look after him or her who hadn't looked after them for a week. I think you've got to do it like that or else the patients might become too dependent on you or you might not get on so well. I think it's just more positive for the patient to be able to change regularly.

The need, at least for some patients, for continuity is illustrated in the following account:

One day you might have certain people to look after and the next day different but the one you had the day before might feel a little bit upset. One of them did yesterday because I was washing somebody else and not them. So I had to *make an effort* [labour required] then when I had finished to go over and talk to him for 20 minutes *because I had nothing else to do* [talking not part of the workload].

The joy of getting through the work as a series of tasks is clearly demonstrated by the following student account:

We worked down one end and everybody was bathed, everybody had their hair washed who wanted to and the ward was absolutely spotless. We were actually getting them bathed without them being told: 'Oh yes you can have a bath; do you really want a bath? Could you have a bath this evening?', and nobody gets a bath in the evening. It's ridiculous. We really felt we had achieved something. The patients were happy and we were happy.

This student was working on Ronda ward at the time and took the opportunity of the sister's day off to organise the work in such a way that she felt she had something to show for her physical rather than emotional labours. Putting patients at the centre of their care was seen by her as time-consuming (and anxiety provoking?) and she believed that everyone was happy partly because the patients had not had to make their own choices but had been fitted into routines.

The ward handovers, written and verbal reports, were also measures of the ward sister's management style and the orientation which underpinned it. In the case of Sister Ronda she used handovers and reports for discussing with each individual nurse the proposed care for the day and then evaluated it with them at the end of the shift. The language used during the handovers on Ronda ward was often very different to that used on the more technically orientated wards.

One student captured the spirit of the ward handovers on Ronda ward when she said:

Sister always stressed talking and it was the things you said rather than what you did . . . like she actually wanted you to describe the content of the conversations you'd had with patients. You couldn't just say words like 'encourage' or 'reassure'. You actually had to say what you'd done to encourage or reassure someone.

I saw evidence of this during fieldwork. One patient began to acquire the label of 'demanding'. You could never walk past her bed without her wanting something: a drink, help to turn over, the commode. She barely said thank you and never smiled. People found her difficult to nurse and would want to avoid walking past her bed. Sister discussed this lady, now in her sixties and a former nurse, during the handovers in order to

92

help students to see why she behaved in this way. They looked at her diagnosis: she had cancer with a very uncertain prognosis; they looked at her family: she was a widow with a number of grown-up children; they looked at her culture: she was Greek and still felt a stranger in Britain, even though she had lived here for over 15 years. The sister spent time talking with the patient about her prognosis, thinking that her 'demands' were probably associated with her anxiety about her future. The students were encouraged to plan the patient's care with her so that she would be able to identify her needs with them in order to pre-empt them rather than 'demand' them.

In contrast, on Edale ward, a technically orientated ward with an emphasis on patients' vital signs, fluid balance and preparation for medical investigations, a student experienced the ward reports in the following way:

> You're not expected to know about people how they feel. I found it difficult in report sometimes. The trained staff would be saying things that I knew about because I'd talked to the patients about them. But they didn't want to know.

This student was a first-warder and felt very much constrained by the hierarchy that did not value her opinion because of her junior status. (This issue is explored further in Chapter 7, where we look at the interaction between the students' individual trajectory and ward management styles.) But, as her colleague, who was currently allocated to Ronda, pointed out: 'That depends on your ward because on Ronda we got as much attention. Everyone, whether you were a first- or third-year'.

To sum up, on Ronda ward the sister's emotional management style was such that both patients and nurses felt valued by her, and as one student said:

> Sister really cares I'm sure. She really does seem to care, so I do too.

Another student thought that what made sister Ronda special was that 'she treats you like a person'. Since the nursing process philosophy and work method expected nurses to treat patients like people the student continued, it was only when the sister treated the nurses like people that the system could work. 'That's the secret of its success on Ronda ward', she concluded.

93

In this chapter I have examined the infrastructure of emotion work on the ward and how the emotional tone is set by the ward sister in a variety of ways. As we saw in the first accounts, her efficiency and competence are enhanced by her positive emotional style.

In the second section we looked at ward sisters' and students' ideal nurses who shared a number of key characteristics similar to those identified by patients in Chapter 2. Both the experienced, pre-nursing process sisters and the students valued a nurse with a 'caring' side, which was synonymous with a people-orientated person. The nursing process then could be regarded as a way of formalising what nurses traditionally regarded as their caring role. Favourable management styles were demonstrated by sisters who were happy, approachable, accessible, valued talking and communication and gave positive feedback.

Sisters organised their work in different ways, motivated by competing rationalities. People-orientated sisters, who corresponded to a nurturing rationality, were more likely to be committed to the nursing process and to recognise and value emotion work than sisters who could be characterised as more medically orientated towards the 'assembly line care of the sick'. Sisters who related to students hierarchically made them feel frightened, anxious and defensive. The students often felt devalued, both as learners and people, and it was those ward sisters who were able to give them back their personhood, which the hierarchy denied, who enabled them to care more for the patients.

When the nurses felt appreciated and supported emotionally by the sisters, they not only had a role model for emotionally explicit patient care but they also felt better able to care for patients in this way. Patients and nurses were sensitive to the ward atmosphere and social relations created by the sister. The assumption is that technical and physical labour are enhanced when underpinned by an emotionally explicit caring style. It was the ward sister's emotional management style that in part answered the student's question as to how possible it was to gear the needs of the institution to 'each person'. The nursing process philosophy and work method created greater emotional involvement for students (which the task allocation method helped them to avoid) and could potentially increase their anxiety.

Overall, however, I found that when a ward sister had an express commitment to the nursing process person-centred philosophy she was more likely to use it as a work method to create the infrastructure which allowed the production and reproduction of emotional labour in her ward.

6 Death and dying in hospital: the ultimate emotional labour[1]

Defining death and dying in hospitals

The impact of dying in hospital and the feelings surrounding its unsuitability as a place to die struck me the first night I did a night shift early on in the study. Hannah and Lily were the regular nurses for the shift. I was there as an extra to help out where I could. Although the ward only had 16 beds, at least half the patients were acutely ill. One patient had been admitted following a drug overdose and was being regularly monitored. Another two were receiving treatment for diabetes. Their blood sugar levels, hovering around danger point, were being constantly checked, and their intravenous infusions regulated.

Then there was Mr Brown, who was dying. We were not aware of it at the time. He was old (87), and advanced cancer had left him weak, emaciated and confused. We had been told by the day staff that he was becoming increasingly 'agitated' (a much used convenience label) and noisy. Would we be sure, therefore, to give him his sleeping tablets and pain killers so that he didn't disturb the other patients?

We started off the night shift as usual, doing the routine tasks. There were the medicines to dispense, a complicated ritual of checking and counterchecking for most of the 16 patients. There were also blood pressures to record and temperatures and pulses to take, not to mention the patient or two who called for the commode or assistance to walk to the bathroom.

Hannah, the staff nurse, asked me to help her with the medicines. When it got to Mr Brown's turn he was in no mood for medicine. He spat most of it out pushing us away. There was no time for coaxing and cajoling. I remember feeling mildly irritated with the wispy haired, cross old man who was determined not to take the medicine. On reflection, fear rather than 'crossness' was the more likely explanation for Mr Brown's behaviour. We left him to finish the drug round, whilst Lily, six months into her training, ran between the other patients, helping with toileting and checking the observations of the acutely ill diabetics and the patient who had overdosed.

Lily and I returned to Mr Brown half an hour later, but by now he was attempting to get out of bed, nightshirt flapping, and still refusing his medicine. We explained that the medicine was to help him sleep, but he didn't seem to understand. Instead, he muttered incoherently, pushing away the spoon containing the medicine and showing unexpected strength for one so frail-looking. I think he thought we might be trying to poison him. It was too late for soothing words, not that either Lily or I felt very calm inside with all the activity and anxiety surrounding the patients with their unstable blood sugars and the man who had taken an overdose beginning to regain consciousness and talk about what he'd done and why.

Finally, Mr Brown, as if worn out with fighting for his life, fell into a fitful sleep. But the anxiety that we felt for the acutely ill patients continued to punctuate the care of Mr Brown all night. We never seemed to have two minutes just to sit with him and calm him and wait with him as he passed from something in between living and dying, a state we were only able to comprehend days later when we returned to the ward to find that he had died. Here was the most profound event of all, and we had not even recognised its imminence in an old man who was strong enough to climb out of bed and push us away. In a ward orientated to acute emergency care and life-threatening situations, Mr Brown's slower, less dramatic, death approached imperceptibly. Our aim that night was to keep him clean and quiet largely for the benefit of the other patients, rather than for his own comfort and safety.

When we found out days later that he was dead we all felt badly; that we had let Mr Brown down. The emotional labour we gave felt unsatisfactory and inadequate for someone who we now realised had been dying.

Feelings about death and dying

When during interviews with students I heard how many of them felt cheated when patients died, I began to understand some of the feelings surrounding Mr Brown's death. The students felt especially cheated if they were off duty when the death occurred. In Mr Brown's case we felt cheated because the last time we had seen him he had been in a distressed state. Some days passed before we were on the ward again, and in the meantime he had deteriorated and died. Consequently we were unable either to improve or to complete the care we had begun.

The students especially felt cheated if the permanent ward staff didn't tell them what had happened to the patient on their return. Not all deaths affected students in this way. But for patients who they had got to know over a period of time and who they felt involved with, being present at their death gave them an opportunity to conclude the care they had begun. For many nurses, closure was attained by performing last offices. I see it as my last duty to them, said one nurse who laid out Mr Owen (aged 50) when treatment for blood cancer finally failed after several weeks in her care.

For those not present at a death, returning to work after a period of absence and not to be told by the trained staff that a patient had died made the students feel doubly cheated. The students believed that the staff's silence represented a failure to recognise the part they had played in the care of the patient and a denial of their right to know that the patient had died. As one student put it 'they just don't want to know'. Another student described the situation in the following way:

On this ward there's a quick turnover of patients and the thing I particularly noticed when I was on nights that you probably nursed someone for all the time you were on the ward. Then you'd go for your nights off and they could have been discharged. You'd return and you wouldn't know that they had gone and you'd ask the trained staff where they'd gone. They'd just say 'well . . . '. Or somebody may have died. Another girl told me she looked after someone for six weeks who died whilst she was on her nights off and she felt cheated that the trained staff hadn't actually told her.

Why did the trained staff seem as if they didn't 'want to know'? One reason was that the students were only allocated to the ward for eight weeks and rarely worked with the same group of staff nurses for any length of time. It was not obvious therefore how the trained staff became aware of how involved students felt about individual patients; nor of their need to know what had happened to those patients whilst they had been away from the ward. Another reason related to the emotional climate of the ward and whether death and dying were explicit components of the work[2]. On such wards it was usual that students and trained staff had contact with each other both informally, during breaks, and formally, during the ward handover, so that there were opportunities for them to discuss their feelings surrounding patients' deaths.

Some of the best managed deaths were those where the trained staff had known the patients and their families over a period of months and sometimes years. Take David, 45, with a heart condition who had been coming to the same ward for three years. Most of the trained staff had known him for at least a year, when a cure still looked hopeful. Now he was coming into hospital for the last time, to die. I observed that the trained staff used certain strategies to manage David's death. Firstly they decided that only trained staff, the people he knew best, should care for him during his final days and hours. His wife was with him throughout this period, supported by the staff who talked with her and helped her with her husband's care. He was moved to the ward's only single room. One staff nurse who willingly took her turn caring for David said that she hoped she would not be on duty when he died because she felt so sad about his impending death. She was unsure how well she would manage her feelings. On this occasion she was not put to the test. David died several hours after she had gone off duty. The ward sister, on the other hand, who had known David during the three years he had been coming to her ward, asked the staff nurses to ring her at home when his condition deteriorated as she wanted to come into the ward to say goodbye. I found this interesting in that the sister was expressing the need to say goodbye to a patient in the same way as the students. But unlike the students she had both the experience and the control over her work to be able to do that.

Death's unpredictability

Some of the difficulties of managing emotions around death and dying in hospital came from its unpredictability. Students expected from the beginning of training to be called upon to nurse dying patients, resuscitate patients following cardiac arrest and to lay out the dead. Students were ever watchful and sometimes fearful that they might be called upon to cope with death in any of these guises, and saw it as part of their training around which they should acquire specific skills. There were no guarantees, however, that they would meet these situations, as a nurse teacher explained:

> You may well have a student who on her night duty on the ward had a death every night. And you'll find another student who's also worked on the ward and not seen a dead patient in three years of training. There are students who have been present at at least three or four cardiac arrests. And others who've passed their final exams and never seen one.

And a student:

> When you're a third-year you're expected to have seen most things and done most things. For example: somebody died and sister said to me 'Well I think you can take care of this now'. Neither me nor another third-year had done last offices before. But we wanted to because we thought 'It's about time'. It just happens. You sometimes miss things like that.

As these two accounts demonstrate, the act of death was more readily identified than the process of dying. Death required clearly defined technical skills. If the patient suffered a cardiac arrest, then resuscitation was required. When the patient was pronounced dead then the body had to be laid out.

The point at which patients were recognised as dying, and the skills required to care for them during their transition from life to death were less easy to define, as shown by our experience with Mr Brown. But what the following incident also showed me was that the training needs of students gave them a functional view of death, which in turn could lead to a fragmentation of the patient's technical and emotional care.

Packaging death

On one of the wards where I had been working, John, a 60-year-old man, lay dying of cancer. He had been admitted to

100

the ward on previous occasions, but none of the staff he knew were on duty. I had been on the night shift a few hours before he died. He lay with a swollen abdomen and restless. We gave him ice cubes to suck and tried to do what we could to make him physically comfortable, but there was no one around who had actually known him in life and it seemed a lonely way to go. I heard later how his death had been managed on the following shift. His care was allocated to two students: one in her final year and the other at the beginning of training. Neither student knew John. The management of the death had the feeling of a neat learning package, partly made possible because the students did not feel any emotional attachment to John. The first-year student had not seen anyone die before and was instructed by the third-year student how it should be done. She was instructed to sit with John and hold his hand. As soon as he had died, two third-year students took over and laid him out, because they 'needed the experience'. I found it interesting to observe how the patient's care, by turning it into a sort of 'learning' package for the students, divided the technical from the emotional labour. Even more than that, the emotional labour had been delegated to the most inexperienced nurse of all, i.e. the first-year student.

Following the patient's death, the first-year student had deferred to two senior students who needed to gain experience in laying people out. She had received some acknowledgement for her labour however, when, shortly after John's death, her seniors had asked her how she was feeling. She said she had felt sad but not upset because she did not know the patient well. On overhearing this conversation, I somehow sensed that she said she felt sad because she felt that sadness was an appropriate feeling to feel[3].

'You knew exactly what to do': a death well managed

Rachel, a student at a similar stage of training, also took part in a patient's death that was managed in a more involving and emotionally explicit way. The patient was a Miss Roberts, in her late eighties. She was slowly recovering from bowel surgery when one morning she woke with excruciating abdominal pain. The doctor was called and X-rays ordered. But there was a long time lapse before she was transferred to the X-ray department and only mild analgesia was given because of the medical tradition of not wanting to 'mask the pain' before finding its cause. Patients who were Miss Roberts' neighbours told me how Rachel cradled Miss Roberts in her arms speaking soothingly to her in an effort to comfort her pain[4].

Miss Roberts was diagnosed as having an inoperable bowel obstruction arising from a postoperative complication. When she returned from having her X-ray she was given stronger pain-killers at last and she lapsed into semi-consciousness. The staff nurse who was on duty came and sat with Rachel, who remained with Miss Roberts until her sister was called. She died some hours later peacefully with her sister and Rachel by her side and a vase of her favourite heavily scented flowers on her locker. She was a devout Catholic, and the priest had given her the last rites before she lapsed into unconsciousness. When she had finally died, the staff nurse asked Rachel if she felt able to help her lay out Miss Roberts. She readily agreed.

I spoke with Rachel and her friend Jill a few days after Miss Robert's death. Rachel said:

I got quite attached to Miss Roberts, but she was old and she had to go sometime. It was sad.

PS.   The other patients told me how much you cared for Miss Roberts on her last day.

R.   Well I just realised that she was in total agony.

J.   You knew exactly what to do. You'd nursed her much more than anybody else. You were her nurse.

R.   I don't know.

J.   You did. I didn't know what to do.

R.   I suppose I looked after her quite a few times.

This short extract illustrates a number of points. Rachel had formed a relationship with Miss Roberts because she had looked after her a number of times. She therefore knew her quite well, to the extent that Jill saw her as *her* (Miss Roberts') nurse. The staff nurse, recognising that Miss Roberts was dying, called her relative and clergyman and supported Rachel to complete her care to its natural conclusion. On this occasion, impending death was recognised and prepared for, and holistic rather than packaged care was given.

The technical and emotional labour of death

In some wards, such as the oncology wards, nurses were regularly confronted with death. They became familiar with the technical aspects of laying people out and overcame some of their fears: 'You get to lay out so many people. You know how to do it. It's gruelling, horrible, but I'm not so afraid of death now'.

But as the student also observed: 'One of the problems on a ward like that is you become so blasé. The staff nurses, it's ruining their careers. The involvement with patients becomes too much and they become hard'.

What the student was describing was a process of emotion management by the nurses to distance themselves from patients and the feelings surrounding their deaths. But, as she saw it, becoming blasé and hard as a defence against involvement was ruining their careers. A patient also made a similar observation. She was a 53-year-old care assistant. I was interviewing her to find out her perspectives on nursing, given some of the similarities with her own occupation. She described herself as 'too emotional' to be a nurse. 'It's like when one of my clients dies, it's like losing one of your own'. She paused and reflected: 'Still, some of the nurses must feel the same. But in those cancer wards they must need to change to prevent getting involved'[5].

The following accounts illustrate why students were concerned with dominating technical skills around the management of death or preventing it, as in the case of cardiac arrest. Night duty was a time when they particularly felt a need for those skills, because it often felt dark and lonely with fewer staff around and patients sleeping.

One student described her first week of night duty on a cancer ward as a junior student. She recounts that she 'hated the whole week of it, but I think I learnt. I think we had two deaths that week and it was quite traumatic, but it built up my confidence'.

Another student, reflecting on her first experience of night duty, said how much she had learnt, particularly when she had witnessed a cardiac arrest. She continued:

103

Until then I was afraid of cardiac arrests. It was also the first one for the third-year I was on duty with. The man died. We were both very upset but because I was the first-year I was sent to supper, but nobody supported the third-year. I learnt from that too that third-years still need support.

These accounts suggest that death and cardiac arrest were events that the students feared, but having experienced them gave them the confidence to handle them technically in the future.

What was less obvious was where and how they learnt to manage their emotions around these events. As the last account illustrates, a third-year student was expected to cope, regardless of how inexperienced and upset she felt following a patient's sudden death from cardiac arrest. The student who had shared the experience with her learnt not only technically from the situation about how to manage a cardiac arrest, but also the importance of dealing with the feelings generated from such a stressful event.

Sister Kinder, who we met in Chapter 5, shows us one way in which students can learn to manage their feelings around such events. Following an emergency on her ward, she called students into the day room and discussed the event with them, in order to find out how they were feeling and to reassure them of a job well done.

Although students were grateful for Sister Kinder's recognition of their needs in this informal way, they were doubtful that managing feelings around death and dying could be formally taught. A common view was that: 'You can't be taught to react . . . if you want to talk about things like death you usually talk about it to your friends when you come off duty'.

Learning about death, like any learning associated with feeling management as expressed in Chapter 3, was seen to be experiential: 'You learn by the way other people do things, like talking to the terminally ill'.

We saw in Chapter 4 that students were more likely to identify 'terminal care of patients and relatives' as a valuable educational experience on the oncology wards compared with the general medical wards. Yet deaths could occur on any of the wards. Indeed, many of the accounts of dying presented above were taken from wards other than oncology wards. On these wards, however, the emphasis was much more likely to be on the patient's technical care. Ward tutorials organised by the nurse tutors also tended to concentrate on patients' diseases and treatment. Generally, students preferred it like that. They regarded talking about feelings and attitudes as a waste of time. Occasionally, they mentioned tutorials which addressed the need to do emotional labour and its cost. When they did, as the student illustrates below, these tutorials played an important part in helping students deal with their feelings.

Yesterday we had a session on the ward with one of the social workers and our tutor. It is very stressful on there because a lot of the patients are young and they are dying of cancer. It was very useful. We could just say what we like and you can realise that it's not just you that feels stressed but probably everyone is feeling the same.

This comment about feeling the same was very important. There was no need for pretence and for being seen to cope when everyone else was feeling the emotion of working in such a stressful environment. The nurses could say how they felt within the confines of the tutorial, allowing them to keep in touch with their feelings when they returned to the public arena.

Death and bereavement

I am now going going to tell two stories about two different patients on two different wards. The stories have some striking similarities. They are stories about elderly patients, both of whom were bereaved of close relatives and one of whom faced his own death. The key people who cared for them were student nurses in their first few months of training. The student nurses were very much in touch with what the patients were going through, but had no arena in which to work on those feelings and emotions.

The first story concerns Mr Lawrence, a man in his eighties. Mr Lawrence was admitted from his local hospital for a palliative procedure to relieve the large tumour in his common bile duct. The tumour was causing a damming up of bile and by the time he was admitted to the ward his skin had turned a profound yellow. Mr Lawrence looked heavy and uncomfort-

105

able. His skin itched from the bile pigments and he complained of nausea and not being able to eat. He looked very miserable and withdrawn. Because he hadn't officially been told of his diagnosis, it was presumed that he didn't know that he had cancer. Judging from his facial expressions and behaviour I doubted somehow that he didn't know. Soon after admission Mr Lawrence's son died suddenly of a heart attack. Mr Lawrence drew in to himself even further, lying silently on his bed with the curtains drawn around him. We were told in the ward report by the trained staff that he did not wish to attend his son's funeral. Again I wondered how much of this was based on assumptions and superficial discussions.

On this ward, it was very much the trained staff who controlled communication and exchange of information. A comment in my field notes during this period reads: 'A very silent exchange: nurses with heads down scribbling; only trained staff giving information. Few comments made by students. For feedback, trained staff asked to be notified of any changes in patients' conditions'.

Not surprisingly, it was difficult to work out from these ward handover reports just how much real assessment of Mr Lawrence's emotional state had taken place.

The trained staff acknowledged in the handover reports that Mr Lawrence was depressed following his son's death. The nurses were instructed to 'chat' to him. There was no discussion or guidance about how to do this and what to say.

When Jane, one of the staff nurses, told me how difficult it was to talk to Mr Lawrence, I began to understand why the students were not being given any better guidance than to 'chat' to him. She explained that whenever she attempted to talk to him he started crying. 'I just avoid him now', she said. Jane was not an unkind person; she just found difficulties talking to people about their feelings. She liked to get on with what she saw as the 'real' work of the ward: the bedbaths, the dressings and the medications. It was interesting that when I left the ward at the end of fieldwork, she thanked me for being an extra pair of hands.

On talking to Lorraine, a first-year student nurse, about Mr Lawrence she told me just how helpless she had felt to support him. After about 12 days in the hospital the doctors decided that as Mr Lawrence did not seem to be making any progress he'd better be transferred back to his local hospital. This was often the pattern with patients who had come from other hospitals for specific treatments. If it looked as if they might die, the doctors made hurried arrangements to get them off the ward. It was as if they did not want to have a patient who had not responded to their treatment dying on them. It was almost as if Mr Lawrence decided that he couldn't face another move. The night following the doctors' decision to transfer him to his home hospital, Mr Lawrence began to vomit blood, and within hours he was dead. That night, Lorraine was on the night shift. This is what she said about him:

> From the moment I nursed him, he just wanted to give up life altogether; he was very apathetic, I'd say. There was nothing you could do. I used to go and sit and talk to him if I had time, but he was just not willing to talk, he wasn't one of those patients who bottled everything up and then came out with it. He just gave one word answers all the time and you felt you weren't getting anywhere and you felt: well, he was eighty or whatever and it's his choice really. I've always heard that people could give up and just turn their backs or whatever, but that's a real classic case.

Lorraine described her efforts to help Mr Lawrence, but to no avail because she felt: 'He was just rejecting me totally, and you felt as if you were imposing on his privacy. He kept the curtains half drawn as well. I always felt this is not my position to come here'.

I knew how she felt. I had had the same feelings when trying to talk to Mr Lawrence myself, as had Jane, the staff nurse who had started avoiding him when every time she talked to him he began to cry. Lorraine had recognised the need to do emotional labour for Mr Lawrence, but had lacked guidance and support on how to manage her feelings and the feelings that he generated.

Lorraine and Jane clearly felt dissatisfied with the way in which they had managed Mr Lawrence's emotional care. Jane withdrew her emotional labour by avoiding him. Lorraine felt rejected, and believed the patient had given up the will to live, so excusing her from 'imposing on his privacy'.

The final story concerns Jill, a student on her first ward. Her work as an au pair with a family where the mother of young children was dying of cancer had prepared her for dealing with issues around death and dying. She was surprised, therefore, on her first placement, a cardiology ward, to find that the ward staff didn't expect her to be interested in people. She said:

> I'm much more interested in the social side of things, making patients happy like Bridget . . . there should be someone who can sort things out for her, sort out what's going round in her head.

Bridget was an elderly patient who had been admitted to the ward when her husband had died suddenly from a stroke. She was suffering from Parkinson's disease and was sometimes forgetful. She had been pronounced 'unable to cope alone at home', since her husband had been the main care giver. I met her on the morning after her admission. She was small and slim with shoulder length hair, a wide friendly mouth and large spectacles. She walked with the shuffling gait typical of Parkinson's disease. Bridget was warm and open and said what she felt. Even though she was 67 years old she had a childlike manner, which probably came from years of being cared for by her husband. They had no children. When she spoke of him, Bridget's eyes filled with tears, saying how good he had been to her and what was she going to do without him. She referred to him as 'daddy'. Many of the students presumed that Bridget was confusing her husband with her father and took this as a sign that she was demented. This wasn't so. Bridget, like many elderly working class couples, especially those without children, referred to their spouse as 'mum' or 'dad'. Bridget was shocked and disorientated by her husband's death, but she wasn't demented.

I noticed that student Jill talked a lot with Bridget. They sat closely together at the end of Bridget's bed talking at some length. Jill was quietly attentive with head inclined and eyes closely focused on Bridget.

There was some confusion about whether Bridget should go to her husband's funeral or not. The general line on the ward was that she did not want to go, but Jill had other opinions, based on her many discussions with Bridget. During the ward report, Jill told me that she had tried to make Bridget's wishes known to the trained staff. They responded by looking surprised at her intervention and turning their attention to the nurse who was in charge of the shift as if seeking more reliable

108

information. In the end Bridget did get to her husband's funeral, but Jill was not satisfied at the way it had been managed. She described the circumstances to me:

I was really quite upset about Bridget's husband's funeral. I found that very frustrating, whisked off at the last minute. I actually said to one of the staff nurses 'She does want to go you know' and she said 'we've asked her and she doesn't'. But I said 'she just told me and she wants to go'. And I thought well I have no say in it. And suddenly there was a great drama and laughs and giggles and she was got off at the last minute in a taxi. It was a mess but I couldn't do anything about it.

As in the case of Mr Lawrence the enormity of bereavement had not been discussed amongst the ward staff. The person who had invested the most emotional labour in helping her to sort out her feelings about going to the funeral was Jill, a first-year student. Jill felt she had been regarded as too junior to be taken seriously by the trained staff and helpless to intervene. Neither had she been allowed to accompany Bridget to the funeral. The staff had finally taken on board that Bridget wanted to go to the funeral, but Jill felt they had handled it badly. They turned their last-minute decision into a 'drama' with laughs and giggles, possibly to hide their own embarrassment as well as to distract attention from the sadness of the occasion.

Bridget's situation is reminiscent of Mr Lawrence's. It was reported that he did not want to go to his son's funeral. Similarly, Bridget was said not to want to go to her husband's funeral. Jill invested emotional labour and elicited an opposite response to the official one. But Bridget welcomed the opportunity to talk about her feelings. Lorraine described the difficulty of caring for Mr Lawrence. Unlike Bridget he was withdrawn and remote. He made Lorraine feel that she was invading on his privacy and was reluctant to talk.

Both these stories illustrate the sensitivity of the first-year students to their own and their patients' feelings. But the feeling rules of the wards were bounded by a rigid nursing hierarchy which operated in two ways. Firstly, it kept the feelings associated with death and dying in place by failing to acknowledge them in the public arena of the ward handovers. Secondly, the trained staff made Lorraine and Jill feel, because of their junior status, that their opinions and views about patients would not be taken seriously.

Both students had important insights on the emotional state of the two patients. In Lorraine's view, Mr Lawrence decided to die. But if her insights had been shared, the way in which he died might have been managed in a more emotionally sustaining way for both nurses and patient. Jill too felt that there was nothing she could have done to avoid the 'mess' surrounding Bridget's husband's funeral. I wondered how long Lorraine and Jill would retain their emotional sensitivity in a hierarchy that neither acknowledged nor sustained it.

The role of the hierarchy in managing death

The hierarchy on many wards kept students and trained staff very separate from each other. They inhabited two different worlds and developed separate sets of social relations with the patients. The trained staff were more likely to get to know and invest in the deaths of the patients that had been coming to their ward over time. The students became involved with patients they had nursed during their eight-week placement. Common to both groups was that nurses did not feel the same way about the death and dying of all their patients but only those with whom they had formed a relationship, usually over time.

The hierarchy also served to separate technical from emotional labour by dictating that, at certain stages of training, students should be able to perform specific technical tasks around death and dying, such as cardiopulmonary resuscitation and last offices.

There was also an expectation that the more senior a student was the more likely she would be expected to cope with upsetting situations. It seemed that because students' feelings were rarely acknowledged in the open arena of the ward that they were likely to develop distancing strategies which kept them from personal involvement. They recognised that, as they progressed through their careers, they might become hard. But they also recognised that if they hardened and distanced too much they would be unable to nurse with feeling.

On the other hand, they were unwilling to believe that they could learn to 'react'. They preferred to see learning about feelings and emotions associated with death and dying as experiential: going through the experiences themselves and observing what other people did. Their reluctance to recognise the skill of learning and how to manage complex feelings was bound up with the way in which death and dying were defined in hospitals according to the patient's diagnosis and the feeling rules of the ward determined by the medical specialty, the hierarchy and the ward sister's work preferences and priorities.

7 The caring trajectory: caring styles and capacity over time

The 'ideal' nurse or ward sister had a 'caring side'. She put people first and organised her work in an emotionally explicit way to make others feel safe and cared for. Not all nurses chose to organise their work in this way, but preferred to focus on tasks and hierarchy which made others feel anxious and defensive. What happened to students' caring styles and capacity to care during their three-year training, and what were the factors that shaped their emotional careers?

First-year students: 'so good to have around'

Students believed that they changed during their training. They came into nursing fresh and enthusiastic, but by the end of three years they had become cynical and disillusioned. They remembered with nostalgia their first year and looked to the current juniors who were 'so good to have around'.

> Nurses do tend to get a bit more cynical as they get used to the job, as they feel more at home. So it is good to have someone more fresh. They are very good at talking to the patients and take a lot of time perhaps because they are not so aware of what is to be done.

Or:

> Too often we just well, we get into a rut of doing something and we just continue to do it because it has to be done and that's the way. Then you get the first-years and they are not so rushed and stressed as you are, and they don't have the responsiblity and that allows them to step back a bit and ask 'why is it done like that?'

112

Another student described the 'uncanny way of getting to know your patients, which you seem to lose. You don't know half the technology which is going on around you. You are unaware of the necessity for speed to get all the jobs done. I used to often get shouted at, well sort of reminded that I had umpteen things to do when I was sitting there talking to patients'.

The first-year students were described in this way because they were still close enough to the beginning of their training to go beyond the medical labels to see the person behind the disease and to see talking to patients in the absence of technical knowledge as a central part of their work. Note how in Chapter 5 'talking' was seen as something to do after the 'real' work had been completed, except for a student at the beginning of training. Similarly, first-year students were 'not so aware' of what else had to be done (besides talking) and would be 'shouted at' or 'reminded' that they had 'umpteen [other] things to do', the 'real' work of bedbaths or tidying the sluice or linen cupboard.

These descriptions of the way in which students change are reminiscent of their changing perspectives on the content of nursing knowledge and practice. We saw in Chapter 3 how students shifted from seeing nursing as 'basics' and 'people' work to the absolute facts of 'diseases, drugs and therapy'. These perspectives are interconnected with their changing feelings about nursing and the loss of getting to know their patients, the acquisition of technical knowledge, and feeling the need 'to get all the jobs done' under perceived pressure from the trained staff.

The following account of a patient in pain, recounted by a student at the end of her first ward allocation, illustrates the 'uncanny way' a new nurse has of getting to know her patients, but who felt unable to persuade the trained staff to institute measures to relieve that pain. She thought that the patient was not being given adequate analgesia to control the pain. I asked her if she could not have used the lunch-time report to make her observations and recommendations known to the trained staff. She was doubtful, feeling that her junior status prevented the trained staff from taking her seriously, but also from seeing the person behind the pain, as she (a new entrant to nursing) still could. Another explanation for their reactions was that, drawing on the third-year accounts, they had 'got into a rut' of always doing things in the same way and feeling rushed and stressed to

113

do the 'real' work which prevented them from stepping back and asking 'why?'. The student, still upset more than a week after leaving the ward, describes the incident from her point of view:

S. Joyce was in agony every time we moved her. If only they had given her something to kill the pain just an hour before we moved her, then it wouldn't be so hard lifting her. That's what she's going to be like for the rest of her life, every day, the same old pain.

Q. Was it not possible to give her painkillers?

S. You could tell the trained staff that the patient wants something, like the painkillers. I even wrote it in the kardex [nursing record]. But they [trained staff] gave the impression that you're not there to tell them what to do. They just thought she was a nuisance.

The student then went on to describe her reactions to what she saw as the trained staff's indifference.

I feel like I want to go out and change things already, like people in pain. What the hell! They're not going to get addicted. You just kill the pain.

I asked her what she meant about the patient 'getting addicted'. She said that she'd noticed that a lot of nurses seemed to be reluctant to give patients too many painkillers because they believed they would get addicted to them. Hayward (1975) reported similar findings in his study of nurses' management of patients' pain, and it is likely the student recalled the research from a recent class. In Joyce's case, the student believed that the trained staff had 'overlooked' the need for pain control because they had not fully understood the extent of her pain.

S. It would have been possible to give her painkillers but they just overlooked it. They just thought she was sitting there normally. Well she was but they didn't realise that every time we moved her she was in terrible pain.

Q. How did you know?

S. Well, we used to take her out of the ward in a wheelchair with her legs down and she was really shaking and I said

114

'Listen, I'll put the leg rest on, that'll be better' and after that we started using it. Nobody seemed to give her painkillers. She was on a lot of tablets, but I don't think they were painkillers. I think the doctors tend to be reluctant about painkillers anyway. It's like curing them without a cure. They think they're going to go downhill. She had Paget's disease which is difficult to cure.

This was perhaps an example of 'assembly line care of the sick' in which, as suggested by the student in Chapter 4, if the patient did not conform to the 'doctor's sort of norm' then they were at 'a loss what to do'. If the ward sisters also subscribed to a similar view of the work then the students were left on their own to deal best with their own preferences and priorities, especially at the beginning of training when they did not have any yardsticks by which to judge the alternatives.

I found many such examples of first-year students investing in patients in a personal way and making a significant contribution to their care. When, for example, students were given some choice over the patients allocated to their care, the first-years, and particularly those on their first ward, chose to care for the same patient, day after day. The first-ward students were more likely than any other group to ensure continuity of care for certain patients. Often these patients were the elderly, chronically sick and physically handicapped, like Joyce described above. Others included Bridget and Miss Roberts in Chapter 6.

Medical intervention and technical procedures were often at a minimum for these patients, and junior students were judged by their seniors to be able to look after patients who 'only' required so-called basic nursing. As students progressed through their training they were more concerned to consolidate their technical and organisational abilities than to look after dependent patients.

The first-ward students, on the other hand, derived security from looking after the same patients over a period of time and consequently got to know them personally. Often because of their age and physical state these patients had many emotional needs that the first ward students were more aware of than any other staff members. But, as the incidents of Joyce and others described elsewhere show, the students' junior status militated against the trained staff recognising their insights and supporting their care. The other problem was that if their insights were not recognised and validated as 'work' the first-year students were not always able to respond therapeutically to their

115

patients' emotional, and in the following case recounted by a tutor, also physical needs.

A student described an incident where 'this patient was vomiting and was therefore unable to go home. And the first ward nurse simply couldn't cope with that. All she could say was "It'll be all right" over and over again'.

The first-ward nurse wanted to be with the patient and comfort her both because she was vomiting and also because of her disappointment at being unable to go home. Her lack of experience in coping with a vomiting patient apparently robbed her of her usual repertoire of reassuring words.

But there was also Miss Roberts' case, described in the previous chapter, where because Rachel, the first-year student, had got to know her over time she was able to give her loving care during her death agony. The staff nurse's sensitive care of both Rachel and Miss Roberts enabled her to do this.

During the second year, the students were allocated to specialist wards. They were often supernumerary and they derived support not only from the trained staff but also from each other. It was during the second year that they were allocated to the psychiatric wards. As I described in Chapter 4, these wards were explicitly geared towards communication and interpersonal skills, and provided the means by which the students learnt to do emotional labour. But they were quickly propelled back into the heady world of the acute general hospital where the predominant management styles packaged both them and their patients and gave them little opportunity to put these skills into practice[1].

Third-year students: 'the blues time'

The third and last year of training was difficult for students. We saw in the last chapter, for example, how they were expected to be able to perform certain tasks by certain stages in their training, irrespective of actual experience, like the ultimate labour of them all described in Chapter 6: managing death and dying. They also felt that juniors got all the 'psychological support' whereas they were expected to 'cope on their own' (see p. 104). We have just seen how they feel responsible for getting 'all the jobs done' and to work 'at speed' which made them feel 'rushed and stressed'. The student, quoted in

116

Chapters 1 and 5, was also a third-year, who felt responsible for taking on the 'whole caring attitude' of the ward if the ward sister failed to do so.

The beginning of the third year was particularly difficult when students put on their red belt, the symbol of their seniority, for the first time. 'People (staff, patients, other students) just look at the belt', one student said 'and fail to realise the difference between someone just at the beginning of their third year or about to take their state finals'. They felt very unconfident to be back in the general wards after nearly a year of specialties where they were not the principal workforce.

A number of students I met or interviewed at the beginning of their third year were feeling disillusioned, unhappy and considering leaving nursing. One student grappling with the decision to leave nursing said:

When I went through the stage of being generally fed up and talked to my friends, you'd be amazed! Some of them said it before I did. But according to one of the tutors it always happens at this stage of training. She called it the 'blues time' because she said 'It's recognised that people are disillusioned and fed up at this stage of nursing'.

The categorisation of extreme feelings in this way 'normalised' them at risk of devaluing the personal difficulties that the student was going through. For this student, it was talking to other students rather than the tutor which swayed her decision to stay in nursing. She said:

When I spoke to some of my friends, I found that it's not just me. It's the place, the job. That's quite an exciting thing to discover that it's not just me.

In a later interview, towards the end of training, the student described the interaction between personal tragedy and trajectory.

You remember, I nearly left. I used to say was it happening just to me or was it happening to everybody? But you know, there were so many negative things happening to me. My father died. And I had so many negative feelings about my work and my colleagues on the ward.

117

Remember, too, the student in Chapter 4 who was allocated at the beginning of her third year to an oncology ward in the wake of her mother's death from cancer. The student felt very distressed by the experience, but neither did she feel she was able to tell anybody about her situation. So she just put up with it, feeling frustrated by patients who wouldn't help themselves and staff who appeared unsympathetic.

Amidst all these feelings and life events, students had to prepare for their state final examinations. This period of training was also categorised by the tutors as a phase when students were described as suffering from 'tunnel vision'. The reason why tutors described them in this way was because the students had one aim in the last months of training: to study as hard as they could in order to pass their final examinations. Given the prescriptive and formulaic format of the examination in the mid-1980s it is hardly surprising that the students reacted in this way.

Personal emotion work

We have seen from the questionnaire data presented in Chapter 4 that students felt comparatively high levels of anxiety and stress from feelings that they were not generally expected either to feel or express (see 'When the feelings don't fit', p. 57). The feeling rules of the City Hospital training were such that they undertook emotion work to suppress these feelings in public.

Students told me about the traumas of starting out on their training, the upheaval of leaving home and taking six months to settle down.

One student said, 'I don't think I learnt much in my first six months as I was *frightened* . . . I don't remember a great deal about it . . . . I think it was because I was *all tensed up*, really'.

A common fear among students was that they would be 'thrown in at the deep end'. This meant that they were fearful of the unknown, such as going to a ward for the first time with nobody to orientate them. I remember one day, when I was working as a participant observer, a brand new first-warder arrived on the ward. The ward was very busy and short-staffed because one of the trained nurses was 'off sick'. The student was frequently left alone with patients as the third-year student who was supposed to orientate her kept unavoidably rushing off

118

with other patients to the operating theatres. Because I was supernumerary and able to fit in around the other nurses, I worked in place of the third-year student, planning and giving patient care with the first-warder. It is impossible to predict what the outcome would have been if I hadn't been on the ward that morning (I wasn't counted on the off duty rota) but there is a good chance that if I hadn't, the student would have felt she had been 'thrown in at the deep end'. As it was she felt relatively overwhelmed at the end of the morning's work.

Students were also apprehensive of night duties with low staffing levels and very sick patients, like the night I spent on Mr Brown's ward (see Chapter 6). They were particularly fearful of their first set of night duty after only six months' training. One student told me how she had spent her first holiday worrying about 'going on nights'.

Students even well into their third year experienced the first few weeks of a new allocation as a very anxious time. One student told me: 'I don't know if anyone really appreciates how anxious you are starting a new ward'. Another student told me that she found it easier to slip into the ward routine as a third-year: 'It used to sometimes take me three or four weeks, especially if there was a difficult staff relationship. Now I feel quite relaxed after about two weeks'. Another third-year student appeared 'really down' during her first few days on the ward according to a first-year, but 'really changed' after she had settled down. I was working as a participant observer on the same ward at the time and also noticed how the third-year student visibly relaxed and smiled more after a week or so. I remember her on her first morning coming up to me and asking rather apologetically (third-year students were supposed to know everything) if I could show her how a catheter leg bag worked, never having seen that particular type of appliance before.

One of the reasons that third-year students felt so anxious was because of the expectations that the ward staff had of them, which in one tutor's view were sometimes 'beyond' them. We saw for example how they were expected to 'cope on their own'. She also summed up the other pressures on them:

> There is the need for them to be able to be in charge and to teach and to appear confident when they don't have any confidence. They don't want to disappoint the juniors, but

they are not given a lot of valuable support themselves because the ward staff think they are third-years and should take responsibility.

A case in point was made in the last chapter, where the third-year students were expected, by virtue of their stage of training rather than actual experience, to take charge in any situation associated with death and dying.

Trained staff also saw the contribution of 'kind and quiet' third-years who 'change the atmosphere' of the ward.

The weight of the nursing hierarchy in dictating students' roles and relationships is evident in the following statement, made to me by a student just beginning her third ward allocation. This was the first time in her training that she had had students junior to herself. She said: 'It's strange when you've actually got someone turning round and asking you something. You're not quite the bottom of the dirt pile anymore'.

Feeling that you are at the bottom of a dirt pile explains the helplessness and frustration that junior felt in influencing patients' care without the support of their seniors.

In Chapter 2, we saw that one way that students learnt to appear confident was through their assessments. The assessments also reinforced their roles and relationships at different stages of their trajectory, so that they felt able to support other students.

Third-year students recognised that they were important to the juniors because: 'We aren't quite so detached as the trained staff. You feel more like the first-years do'.

Another student said: 'You forget how as a first-year you are frightened of approaching anybody more senior than you'.

This observation is illustrated by the following incident, recounted by a senior third-year student who took on the responsibility for having a word with a first-year student who was too frightened to address the ward sister directly.

Sister was standing next to me during the drug round and a first-year student came up to me and said 'Could you tell sister that Mr Green's temperature has gone up?' Well [laughing] Sister, she just died! She said 'I think she's a bit scared to talk to me don't you?' so I thought, 'I had better have a word and say "well, sister won't bite you!"'. But then there must be some kind of awe still for the first-years. I mean I remember feeling frightened of the sister when I first started training, but you forget quite easily.

This incident illustrates the power of the hierarchy in provoking feelings of fear in a student (at the bottom of the dirt pile) to the extent that she felt unable to address the ward sister face to face, but had to go through an intermediary. It also illustrates the responsibility the third-year student felt to act as an intermediary on behalf of the junior student.

The responsibility felt by another third-year student towards a first-year is demonstrated in another account. The senior student described how, despite finding herself in a very frightening situation, she had consciously suppressed her own feelings in order to protect a first-year student:

I had a busy set of nights on the second ward in my third year. That was quite frightening in that we had a lady who kept obstructing her breathing, and to begin with I really panicked. But then there was me and a third-warder and I thought 'God! if I panic then what will she do?' That finally made me sort myself out and there were a lot of different things to be done. And I thought after that well I didn't need to panic so much.

But there was also the perspective that you had to do emotion work on yourself in order to deal with the hierarchy and your fear of it. One student told me:

I found that it's up to you to brave the initial fear of a trained staff uniform and ask questions. If that staff member re-members what it's like to be a first-year nurse then your individuality is preserved.

Caring factors

What then were the factors that influenced the students' caring styles and capacity during their three-year trajectory and their choice of future emotional styles?

Ward management styles: recognising or repressing individuality

We saw in Chapter 5 how ward sisters' management styles could be characterised according to whether they managed their wards through hierarchy and tasks as part of the 'assembly line care of the sick' or by 'nurturing' people. Students found themselves caught between these competing management styles as they moved from ward to ward. During any one allocation, the extent to which a sister's ward management style recognised or repressed a student's individuality (i.e. a style that nurtured people or managed tasks) emerged as an important factor in the caring trajectory. The importance of recognising a student's individuality has already been suggested by the student's comment above who describes the importance of the trained staff remembering 'what it's like to be a first-year'. It is more likely that students will be able to approach ward sisters who are committed to people, rather than hierarchy and tasks, and that these sisters will remember their own feelings as junior nurses.

The importance of management styles in recognising or repressing a student's individuality are described by a nurse tutor in the following way:

Every ward operates in its own way. It's a culture shock. Some wards encourage the students as individuals and others repress it. It varies with the individual as to what happens when they go to the ward.

Every eight weeks the students were required to adjust their preferences and priorities to individual styles of management that either encouraged or repressed their individuality.

But the tutor also described how different students perceived their ward experiences differently. She said: 'It's fascinating to see their reactions, because you can have two people sitting there and you don't know they're talking about the same ward'. When I asked the tutor why she thought students reacted so differently, she said: 'It's their personality, expectations, what they've heard on the grapevine and whether the individual style of management suits them'.

When we consider the mechanisms and motivations that bring trained staff and students together at different stages of their trajectory we can begin to see how the students' own caring styles and capacity might be either reinforced or discouraged by particular management styles over time. Because of their experiences on particular wards at particular times, they began to form their own preferences and priorities for their future work and to decide which 'style of management suits'.

The sisters and staff nurses who had chosen to work together formed a cohesive group which supported a particular philosophy and style. Students, on the other hand, had little say over their ward placements and were allocated for an eight-week period to fulfil their training requirements and the staffing needs of the hospital. Because of the functional way in which their allocations were planned, some students found themselves in intolerable situations, like the student who didn't want to be on an oncology ward because her mother had recently died of cancer, but felt unable to say anything about it.

Unless students were on wards like Ronda, where the sister recognised, articulated and supported emotional care, the students found difficulties in resisting the pressures imposed upon them by hierarchical relationships to take on the preferences and work priorities of the ward, rather than maintain their own. In this way, the ward hierarchy could be seen as one of the mechanisms for shaping a student's emotional labour.

Junior students were conscious that the ward hierarchy made them 'vulnerable' and 'on the side of the patient'. They were more likely to start out seeing things from the patient's rather than the staff's perspective. The staff nurses might regard patients as 'awkward' and 'up to their old tricks' rather than looking for reasons for their behaviour. Students were less willing to accept labels and stereotypes, but they also found difficulty in resisting the opinions of their hierarchical superiors as the 'experts'. Even when students disagreed with the ward staff's opinions on patients and their care, hierarchical management styles prevented them from either offering alternative perspectives or feeling they could offer such alternatives. The first-year student who cared for Joyce, described at the beginning of this chapter, offers one such example. Although she had found her own ways of relieving Joyce's pain she also felt unable to challenge the staff's view of Joyce as 'a nuisance'.

The issue of hierarchy as a mechanism for shaping emotional labour for more senior students also arises from the critical incident described in Chapter 3. The student, commenting on the incident, observed that her fellow student, also a third-year, 'knew she didn't do what she should have done as a nurse' by convincing a distraught relative to take her psychiatrically disturbed brother home because the medical and trained staff wanted him out of their ward. The pressures put on the student to conform to the wishes of those higher up in the hierarchy made it very difficult for her to maintain her own person-orientated perspective, and she found herself undertaking emotional labour to satisfy the wishes of those in authority rather than to do 'what she should have done' which was to insist that the patient stayed in hospital.

We saw how Sister Ronda would not accept labels and stereotypes, using the ward handover report to explore why students thought patients were behaving in certain ways. She also sought students' opinions and perceptions on patients and their care.

We saw, however, that some students, particularly the third-years who had been exposed to task-orientated nursing and hierarchically managed wards over the years, were resistant to Sister Ronda's preferences and priorities: like the student who found that patient allocation 'went too far'.

I remember another incident during participant observation when a third-year student disagreed with the sister's decision not to sedate a patient with dementia during the day. The patient was quite noisy and tried to get up from her chair to stagger unsteadily around the ward. The student objected on three counts. The patient was disruptive to other patients; she might fall and hurt herself; and she was more difficult to nurse in that she had to be related to. This third consideration was the sister's intention, since she wanted the students to interact with the patient in order to make her feel safe and cared for rather than drugged and remote. The third-year student would fume in the sluice, feeling that she had 'better' things to do. She was having to do emotional labour (suppress feelings in private) in order to present her calm City nurse exterior to the external world of the ward. The difference between Sister Ronda and many other sisters was that she would listen to the student's point of view. For the student however, this did not help as she did not agree with the sister's preferences and priorities, having now formed her own. She was looking forward to the end of her training, when she hoped to become a staff nurse on a surgical ward where the work was organised in a more task-orientated and hierarchical way.

124

Much of the third-year students' resistance to patient involvement and allocation on a regular basis was a departure from the first-year students' choice to invest in patients in a personal way. One explanation for this change, suggested by the third-year student accounts at the beginning of this chapter, was that the juniors had not yet been socialised into caring for patients as if they were on the medical assembly line, but still retained their people-orientated perspective. Since continuous patient allocation was not encouraged and supported on many wards, they quickly moved away from this way of working to taking on the technical and management skills expected of more senior students.

Ward management styles: recognising the student's learning role

Recognition of the student's learning role was another factor associated with management styles that helped students to feel that they were being recognised as individuals. Third-year students warned me when I distributed the ward learning environment questionnaires that I could expect lower scores from them because they felt less positive than the first-years about their training. When I analysed the questionnaire scores I did indeed find that the first-year students' average ratings for the ward learning environment were generally higher than later in training (Tables E12–E15 in Appendix E). I put this down to the cynicism and disillusion that the third-years complained of and their resentment at being used as 'pairs of hands'.

It follows therefore that when ward sisters recognised the students' learning role they felt valued and better equipped to care for patients. Sister Edale, for example, whose ward got top scores, clearly articulated the relationship between teaching students and ensuring patients got good care.

One student explained the importance of a management style that also recognised the student's learning role in the following way:

When you go to a ward the extent to which you *enjoy* the experience, isn't related to the sort of nursing you are doing [i.e. the ward specialty]. It's much more what the atmosphere of the ward is like and *who you are working with*. I think where there is a lot of input from ward staff and they want to teach you, you get a lot more from it and you're *happier* about nursing the patients because you've got more information.

This student articulates the relationship between the trained staff's express commitment to teaching as part of creating the 'caring' atmosphere, the importance of good working relations and the generation of positive feelings: enjoyment and happiness associated with having more information about nursing the patients. I am inferring that a student who enjoys a clinical placement and feels happier is less likely to feel stress and anxiety. I now present four short case studies to illustrate the different ways in which the ward sisters recognised the student's learning role and created the ward learning environment. These case studies are based on participant observation and the questionnaire findings presented in Appendix E.

Recognising the student's learning role: creating the learning environment on four wards

The recognition of the learning role and creation of the learning environment was handled in different ways in each study ward. On Edale, the learning environment was created by a ward sister who prioritised formal ward teaching. The ward specialty (cardiology) was one that generated technical nursing which was readily identified by students as learning material. The workload was described as 'light' and the staffing levels as adequate. Stress ratings were low for this ward. Findings suggested that students experienced stress and anxiety associated with the way in which trained staff handled feedback and expected third-year students to manage the ward. It is possible that these feelings were reduced because of the ward sister's explicit commitment to ward teaching which fulfilled students' expectations for learning. Sister Edale corresponded to the ward sister who was student-orientated and made ward teaching a reality[2].

Sister Windermere expected students to take responsibility for their own learning and patient care. Students were given work orders during handover reports, but were not expected to exchange information and ideas about patient care at the handover report. Formal teaching was not a priority. The nature of the work was readily identified as learning material by students because of the 'variety' and technical needs of patients admitted to Windermere ward. Trained staff involved themselves in patient care which made them physically accessible to the students when they needed advice. Stress ratings for the ward were low. The physical accessibility of trained staff may have helped to alleviate students' feelings of stress and anxiety. Findings suggest that the third-year students found the sister more approachable than first-year students.

The ward learning environment was created on Kinder ward by a sister who prioritised formal teaching and supervising students' care to patients. Students recognised the sister's commitment to teaching, but found her management style created stress. Their feelings of stress were reflected in Kinder's top stress rating. Students also experienced stress from the acute nature of the work on Kinder ward, but they also readily identified emergency patient care as learning material. The high stress ratings on Kinder ward are an interesting finding when compared with the low stress ratings on Edale, where students expected to be stressed from patients having cardiac arrests. Contrary to expectations this was not the case, despite it being a specialist cardiology ward.

The differences in the stress ratings for the two wards with an explicit commitment to teaching appeared to be partly accounted for by the sisters' differences in management style. On Kinder ward, third-year students in particular resented being supervised by trained staff and wanted to take more responsibility for the ward. Third-year students on Edale experienced the opposite situation, feeling that on occasions they were given too much responsibility for managing the ward. But this feeling was not strong enough to militate against students' overall perception of a favourable environment.

Ronda ward rated less highly as a learning environment than the other three wards. The students perceived the learning potential of the ward as low because of the large patient population of dependent elderly. The sister's commitment to the nursing process and communication skills was recognised but not automatically identified as learning material. The heavy workload, coupled with the low staffing levels and lack of trained staff, militated against the provision of formal teaching and supervision. The sister was well recognised by students for her approachable and accessible management style and her concern for their emotional needs. The high stress ratings therefore appeared to be associated with the heavy physical

127

workload, inadequate staffing levels and the lack of trained staff. Some students found the sister's management style too 'unstructured'[3].

In spite of the perceived differences in management style and nature of the learning material on the four wards, the scores obtained for 'provision of learning opportunities' were only statistically significantly higher on Edale, the 'top' teaching ward. The critical variables which interacted to effect this choice were the provision of formal teaching, a ward specialty that was medically and technically orientated and a management style that showed a 'moderate structure'[4].

The ratings for item 2 of the questionnaire 'I am happy with the experience I had on this ward' were relatively favourable for all the wards and no one score showed a statistically significant difference from the others (see Table E16, Appendix E). These findings suggest that the perceived differences in the learning environment of the four wards did not make the students feel any less happy. It is likely that different student preferences and different ward factors interacted to produce their overall perceptions of happiness on each ward.

Personal support

The recognition of their learning role was one important way in which students felt supported. But, in general, they were incredulous at the lack of support they got throughout their training from either their teachers or their ward sisters. They felt that there was no one person who was there for them as an individual. It is little wonder that they talked about becoming cynical in the so-called 'caring profession' that didn't demonstrate any care of its most junior and largest group of carers. One student admitted that 'if you wanted support the tutors would give it, but because there's no opportunity to build up a relationship with them, they're like strangers'. The student was emphasising the importance she attached to good personal relationships, which depended on getting to know someone.

One student said: 'Third-years support first-years on some wards but everyone needs it, as well as reassurance. The third-years get cross at not getting support. Third-years are just expected to cope'.

We noted in Chapter 5 that what made Sister Ronda special was that she gave support and reassurance to everyone, irrespective of stage of training. She was seeing the person first rather than the first-, second- or third-year label and associated expectations. She also recognised and took seriously the students' contribution to care, irrespective of position in the hierarchy.

I also observed that Sister Windermere played a vital role in supporting a third-year student going through the so-called 'blues time'. She noticed how unhappy she looked whilst allocated to her ward. She called the student into her office during a quiet period on the evening shift in order find out the cause of her unhappiness. She was able to talk her through some of her difficulties and discouraged her from leaving nursing at that late stage in her training. The student concluded that: 'I was going through a period of wanting to leave nursing whilst I was on Windermere ward, but sister recognised this and was very supportive through a difficult period'.

If students felt psychologically supported throughout their training then they were more likely to sustain caring styles and capacities that recognised and valued emotional labour as part of their work. What emerges is the importance of the third-year students in the production and reproduction of emotional labour, not only in relation to the patients and the smooth running of the ward, but principally in supporting the junior students.

Coda

The complexity of the caring–learning relationships in which a student finds herself on her trajectory are graphically expressed by a third-year student:

In nursing you have got so many relationships to form with people who you have never met before, who you probably don't like, you may not like out of work, under circumstances that are tremendously difficult. Often the relationships are short and sharp with hierarchy and authority and discipline somewhere mixed up into them, the learning situation as well. And the student who is trying to gain knowledge from this person, who she is trying to form a relationship with, when you add all that together, well I think you are bound to have chaos and I think you do have chaos. And so I think that in the nursing world as a whole everybody moulds everybody else.

129

This student is saying many things of relevance to our analysis of emotional labour. Firstly, she is drawing attention to the central issue of personal relationships in nursing. Many times during this and previous chapters we have been drawn to their centrality in caring and feeling cared for. Often nurses find themselves working with people who they do not like (both patients and other nurses), but they feel they have to suppress these feelings. Often these relationships are short and sharp, because students are constantly changing wards and most patients are 'just passing through'. The shift systems are such that contact between staff, students and patients tends to be fragmented and to lack continuity, even on wards where the nursing process is practised. We saw in Chapter 6 how students could be away from the ward for over a week after a spell of night duty, and thus find that patients whom they had cared for had either died or been discharged.

This student also draws attention to the importance of hierarchy, authority and discipline in shaping these relationships. We saw above how certain management styles and the assessment system could repress rather than encourage a student in her efforts to sustain an individual commitment to caring. We can speculate that if the student is repressed too often for too long in her trajectory, coupled with the need to suppress her own personal feelings, then it is more likely that she will choose hierarchical relationships, labelling and stereotypes as the preferred form of emotional labour by the end of her trajectory.

The student also reminds us that student nurses not only choose nursing to be able to care, but also to learn to care. The importance of relationship work is again raised. The student describes the outcome of the competing demands as 'chaos'. Why is this? My conclusion, from talking extensively with students and experiencing their world, is that this is because there is no single person who they feel is responsible for them; who they can relate to throughout their three-year training and give them feedback on their work. They were incredulous of the lack of support they got except from each other and the occasional ward sister. At every stage of their training they were suppressing their own feelings (i.e. doing emotion work) in order to please others, either their hierarchical superiors or the patients. In this context, the student talks about 'everybody moulding everybody else', a concept that was used by both students and patients in Chapter 2 to describe how nurses became emotional labourers.

In this chapter, as we look at the issue from the point of view of the trajectory, we begin to see that if the student is constantly exposed to 'circumstances that are tremendously difficult', which I would interpret as a lack of caring factors, she will either choose to leave or to develop styles and strategies to protect her emotions.

Emotional labour: styles and strategies

Thus, in order to deal with such extreme feelings nurses developed certain strategies. From the cases referred to in this chapter and described elsewhere in the book, these included various 'distancing' strategies such as developing a 'seen it all before attitude' which made it easier to label patients and their behaviour. Thus by slotting patients into convenient categories such as 'difficult', 'awkward', 'a pain' or 'a nuisance', and projecting images and assumptions upon them associated with their gender, class and race, as described in Chapter 4, nurses were able to 'objectify' them and their symptoms.

The students' discussion of death and dying in Chapter 6 suggested that repeated confrontation with death and laying people out on an oncology ward made even the students 'blasé', after only an eight-week allocation. The students reasoned that prolonged exposure to continual death and dying made the permanent staff appear 'hard' in an attempt to distance themselves from their feelings, in a reverse form of emotional labour. When students returned from their days off wanting to find out what had happened to the patients they had cared for on night duty, they found that 'the trained staff just didn't want to know'. Or take the staff nurse who had to walk away from Mr Lawrence because she found his crying every time she talked to him too difficult to cope with. The staff nurses on Bridget's ward found that the best way they could handle her bereavement was to send her off in a taxi to her husband's funeral at the last minute amidst laughs and giggles. On many wards, the trained staff physically removed themselves from patient and even student contact by going to their offices.

The way in which nursing was traditionally organised around tasks reduced close nurse–patient encounter and reduced anxiety[5]. Even though the nursing process had been introduced to encourage nurses to care for patients rather than to carry out tasks, most ward sisters operated a system that allowed students some choice over the patients they cared for. With the exception of students at the beginning of training, they were likely to change their allocation daily, which permitted them to regulate their personal involvement with patients.

Evidence suggests that these strategies were developed during the caring trajectory if students were repeatedly exposed to a range of emotionally demanding experiences without the support of their hierarchical superiors. Joining 'the other side' in labelling and stereotyping patients was one way of reducing the conflict between their commitment to care and the prevailing ward philosophy and style.

Even a first-warder after only eight weeks on a ward told me: 'It's good to stop and think about how people feel, otherwise you treat them like objects'. Or consider a third-year student who said that: 'It is very hard to appreciate how patients actually feel about what is wrong with them unless you talk to them'.

At this point we remember the haunting words of the first-year student who said: 'if people don't matter then you can't do nursing', a theme that returns again and again. Similarly, a student nearing the end of her training uttered similar words, but with a qualification. She said, 'I came into nursing to care for people. I expected to care for them in pain and when they were dying. What I didn't expect was that the system doesn't always let me do it in the way I want to'.

Students were more likely to feel this way on wards where the sisters managed hierarchically and produced a negative emotional labour which made nurses feel frightened, anxious and stressed.

The divisiveness of the hierarchy was apparent in the way in which it separated the trained staff from the students and transformed them into pairs of hands for performing tasks rather than patient-centred care.

The formal content of their training gave them little guidance on managing complex feelings or on offering a viable alternative to the biomedical base of nursing. They also received little personal support throughout their training from either teachers or ward sisters. But there were also many Sister Rondas, who showed that it is possible to maintain caring styles and capacity over time and to reproduce the nurse with 'the caring side' from one generation to the next. The principal variable was feeling cared for themselves and supported, which allowed the nurses to care more for each other and the patients. The recognition of nursing as people work was at the crux, which made emotional care visible and valued in both the form and content of their training[6].

In this chapter, I have looked at the ways student nurses describe their three-year trajectory from 'freshness' and 'an uncanny way of getting to know their patients' to cynicism and disillusion. The first-year students were still free of technical knowledge and sufficently people-orientated to go beyond the medical labels of the wards.

First-year students invested in patients in a personal way and made a significant contribution to their care. When given the choice they often opted to care for patients on a daily basis. Many of these patients were often seen as 'only' requiring basic nursing and hence within the scope of a first-year student. As students progressed through their trajectory their expectations for nursing changed. They became more concerned to consolidate their technical and managerial skills, but were also expected to take on organisational and other responsibilities, irrespective of their previous experiences, by trained staff.

Third-year students underwent a stressful period known locally as the 'blues time'. It was during that period that a number of students grappled with the decision of whether to leave nursing or not.

Throughout their three-year programme nurses experienced a range of emotions associated with both their personal and training trajectory. They received little formal support and undertook emotional labour to conceal these feelings from the outside world.

The nursing hierarchy dictated students' roles and relationships, and the importance of the assessments in building up their confidence to stick up for each other once more becomes apparent. Third-year students were particularly important in their support of junior students and many of them undertook emotional labour to make them feel safe and cared for. Another perspective emerged: that of the students having to work on themselves to 'brave' the hierarchy.

A number of caring factors were identified which influenced students' caring styles and capacities over time and their personal choice of future forms of emotional labour. Of critical importance was the ward sister's management style in encouraging or repressing students' individuality throughout the trajectory. The nursing hierarchy played an important role in shaping emotional labour and the students' capacity to care throughout their trajectory.

The recognition of the students' learning role by the ward sister was also identified as an important caring factor. The different ways in which the ward sister created the learning environment are described in four short case studies based on participant observation and questionnaire findings.

Personal support given to students was *ad hoc* and depended on the ward sister's management style rather than teachers in the school of nursing.

Finally, the complexity of the caring–learning relationship is described, drawing on the analysis of an extract from an in-depth interview with a third-year student. The fragmentation of personal relationships between nurses and between nurses and patients is described. I speculate that if students' individuality and caring commitment is repressed too often and for too long during the trajectory, coupled with the need to suppress their own personal feelings, then it is likely that they will chose hierarchical relations, stereotyping and labelling as preferred forms of emotional labour by the end of the trajectory.

Unless students were supported by their teachers and ward sisters, they developed styles and strategies which enabled them to distance themselves from patients to protect their own feelings in a reverse form of emotional labour.

But there were also ward sisters with management styles that showed that the critical variable which allowed nurses to maintain 'a caring side' and to reproduce it from one generation to the next was feeling cared for themselves. This required the recognition of nursing as predominantly people work which made emotional care visible and valued in both the form and content of their training.

A number of important questions emerge from these findings which I shall explore in the final chapter.

8 Conclusions

Early readers of my manuscript experienced its content as 'a voyage of discovery', a quest for understanding of what lay at the heart of nursing. Their comments accurately reflect not only what the research was about, but how I went about it. I wanted to discover, through the data, what learning to care meant to students in terms of both its content and process. The preceding chapters have been written in the spirit of that discovery in order to draw conclusions on the meaning of care, its interpretation and transmission in ward and classroom and its effects on nurses and patients. I now summarise my main conclusions.

Concepts of care and emotional labour

Care as a concept is complex. It is referred to on a number of different levels. Nursing leaders exhort nurses to care, but their definitions are limited because they fail to take into account the emotional complexity of caring. Neither do they consider the way in which care is stereotyped as women's 'natural' work nor the gender division of labour and the power relations between doctors (predominantly men) and nurses (predominantly women) within the health service which marginalise care to 'the little things'.

Care is an important notion for nurses and patients. They see it as the essential ingredient of the 'good' nurse and use it to refer to the emotional component of nursing which underpins her technical and physical activities. Student nurses felt better able to care for patients when they felt cared for themselves by the trained ward staff and their teachers. Because care was such a marginalised activity and conceptually ill-defined, I wanted to use the data to re-define it. The accounts of caring from both students and patients suggest that 'caring' does not come

135

naturally. Nurses have to work emotionally on themselves in order to appear to care, irrespective of how they personally feel about themselves, individual patients, their conditions and circumstances. They can also be taught to manage their feelings more effectively.

These data fitted the definition of emotional labour elaborated by Arlie Hochschild (1983), whose work I discovered well into my data collection. I had not started out with the notion of care as emotional labour, but my data led me to select an appropriate framework. I then put Arlie's definition and analysis of emotional labour to the test each time I asked questions of my data. In this way I was able to assess its theoretical viability in the context of nursing. I was interested to find therefore that James (1986) had chosen to combine the two terms in her research, by referring to nursing the dying as 'carework'. The importance of defining care as work cannot be underestimated if this most essential ingredient of what nurses do is to be recognised and valued. But recognition and value are not enough. Care must be supported educationally and organisationally in the institutions where nurses work and learn and by the political and economic structures within society (Tronto, 1987).

The gendered nature of nursing work and the perpetuation and predominance of the Nightingale image are examined in Chapter 2. These findings are of particular interest to recruitment officers at national and institutional level. With a falling population of 18-year-old women from which student nurses were traditionally recruited and a declining interest in nursing as a career, the nurses in my study may fast be disappearing as a distinct group. One important question is whether the predominant image of nursing as women's traditional work will have to change. Evidence from current recruitment literature and posters suggests recruiters recognise that it does. The technical aspects of nursing are given a higher profile and men and older women are targeted as potential recruits (Department of Health, 1990).

At what cost care?

A recent recruitment poster gives a double message: nursing offers two sorts of rewards, emotional and financial. But is the emotional component of caring adequately recognised and remunerated? I suggested in Chapter 1 that it was not. Health planners and managers of the new look health service may be so concerned with fine tuning their budgets that nurses will find themselves with increasing workloads that leave them with little time to do anything but meet patients' physical and technical needs. Emotional care is not easily costed, and may be in danger of being marginalised even further as health care moves to the market place.

Ironically, some private health insurance schemes advertise their services through images of smiling nurses, but without paying them any extra for the emotional component of care. Until the current recruitment crisis, the issue of nurses' pay was not seen as important. In the teaching hospitals there were always more than enough young female applicants willing to work for low wages. Even so, despite being recruited in Nightingale's image the City nurses resented being seen by patients as 'angels' and vocationally motivated. Most of them saw themselves as workers who were doing a job.

The future of nursing theory and practice

The introduction of the clinical career structure during 1988 provided the potential to reward nurses' clinical skills and responsibilities. All nurses, representing half a million jobs, were re-graded over a period of six months. The grading exercise was linked to the annual pay award. In the event, the cost far exceeded the Department of Health's estimations. Although extra monies were made available, local funding had already been allocated. Consequently, many nurses were disappointed with their grading and often found themselves competing with colleagues for a limited number of posts. Despite the difficulties, however, the re-grading process has shown the potential for rewarding nurses for their expertise and improving their career structure (Beardshaw and Robinson, 1990).

The introduction of the clinical career structure is closely associated with the planned reforms for nurse education set out in the UKCC's Project 2000 (UKCC, 1986). Thus, the three-year hospital based programme described in this study, during which students spent the majority of their time on the wards as the principal workforce and only 30 weeks in the classroom, is giving way to American style college programmes and supernumerary clinical status.

But what is the situation in the USA, where many of the educational changes envisaged by Project 2000 have already been implemented? The answer is an acute nursing shortage and falling college rolls. Part of this shortage is associated with high-cost private health care, in which the insurance companies refuse to pay for anything but the most acute phases of illness and many nurses are finding it increasingly difficult to give the level of patient care they desire (Huey, 1988). Hospital administrators looking for ways of making financial savings may be inclined to cut nursing posts. As one leading nurse wrote in a recent US government report 'The value of nursing derives from the content of its work. Nurses care for those who cannot care for themselves; such compassion is a hallmark of civilised society . . . there is a consensus that care should be given when it is needed. But we hate to pay for it . . . and have avoided paying for the real cost of our nursing services' (Lynaugh, 1988). The Dean of one of the most prestigious nursing schools describes the nursing shortage as a 'women's issue' in that nursing (the percentage of female nurses is even greater than in Britain at 97 per cent) provides a caring function which is 'very undervalued by our society' (Sullivan, 1989). The American experience suggests that private health care and changes in nurse education have done little to affect society's perceptions of nurses and nursing.

But what about the nurses themselves? Many of them, as the biggest occupational group within the US health care system, are voicing their dissatisfaction through strike action which appears to be about pay but also about conditions. Nurses complain that they are finding it increasingly difficult to give the level of patient care they desire. These strikes occur in pockets across the country. In September 1989, for example, the nurses from the Oakland Children's Hospital in California were on strike for over two months. The reasons for taking strike action were many, but one important issue emerges pertinent to our discussion on the remuneration of emotional labour. The nurses wanted special duty payment for the added responsibility of caring for children, who they alleged are often more physically and *emotionally* demanding than adults (Lynch, 1989). The nurses also stated that they were taking strike action to 'address a nationwide nursing shortage' which was pushing them all to their physical and emotional limits.

British nurses are expressing similar concerns, as revealed by a recent survey which investigated factors affecting recruitment and retention (Price Waterhouse, 1988). Respondents were particularly dissatisfied with low staffing levels, heavy workloads and inadequate standards of care.

The application of my findings is of particular relevance to the content and form of the new style training, with its emphasis on people and health rather than patients and disease. Findings presented in Chapters 3 and 4 offer important perspectives on the knowledge base of nursing as 'people work' and its relationship between ward and classroom. They show, for example, how nurses define the physical, technical and emotional components of their clinical work according to medical specialties and attach importance to 'liking' some patients more than others. The findings also show that students frequently found themselves in emotionally charged situations which went beyond the medical and technical definitions of their training and back to nursing as 'people work', in which they frequently engaged in emotional labour. Often they experienced anxiety and stress because their emotional labour went largely unrecognised and undervalued as part of 'real' nursing. Neither was it incorporated into the theoretical and practical organisation of their training.

On the basis of these findings I suggest that the emotional components of caring require formal and systematic training to manage feelings, grounded in a theoretical base such as psychology, sociology and the acquisition of complex interpersonal skills. In this way emotion work will be made visible and valued in its own right and not viewed as *just* part of the package of womens' work.

Nurse academics are also proposing nursing theories that go beyond the conceptual limitations of the nursing process. These developments hold possibilities for using research findings from studies such as mine to build an empirically tested knowledge base rooted in practice.

The UKCC's Project 2000 is committed to preparing practioners who are 'knowledgeable doers' and to teach students 'how to learn and how to analyse, to give them confidence and the motivation and facilities to develop themselves in relation to a changing environment' (UKCC, 1985, p.21). These recommendations encourage nurses to re-examine traditional definitions of nursing knowledge, teaching and learning based on notions of tacit knowledge which is uncodified and transmitted through tone, feel and expression (Collins, 1974; Eraut, 1985, p.119). These approaches are more appropriate to recognising emotional

139

labour as a key component of nursing, requiring the acquisition of a set of hitherto uncodified skills.

The importance of integrating intuitive insights with systematic knowledge is being increasingly recognised (Sheehan, 1983). Benner (1984) suggests ways in which a nurse moves through five stages from 'novice' to 'expert'. The use of intuition in decision-making distinguishes the 'expert' nurse practitioner from the beginner. In later writings, Benner and others describe how intuition is developed through and used in clinical practice:

> It is the unique, remarkable capacity of the body to cope with vague, 'fuzzy' information and regions of influence and tension that makes possible the human capacity to function in ambiguous, underdetermined situations (Benner and Wrubel, 1989, p.53).

The findings presented in Chapter 5 are of key importance in understanding emotional labour as part of the labour process of nursing and the conditions necessary to its production and reproduction in the workplace. When nurses felt appreciated and supported emotionally by the sisters, they not only had a role model for emotionally explicit patient care but they also felt better able to care for patients in this way. Patients and nurses were sensitive to the ward atmosphere and social relations created by the sister. The assumption is that technical and physical labour are enhanced when underpinned by an emotionally explicit caring style.

The nursing process philosophy and work method created greater emotional involvement for students than task allocation. It also potentially increased their anxiety.

This finding is of particular relevance given the move across the country as part of the 'New Nursing' to introduce primary nursing which goes beyond the recommendations of the nursing process in promoting continuity of care (Pearson, 1988; Salvage, 1990). Primary nursing further raises the profile of emotional care by placing even greater emphasis on the interpersonal relationship between nurses and individual patients. The need for supervision as used by psychiatric nurses and social workers is being promoted by some primary nurses (Johns, 1990).

In wards where the ward sister had an express commitment to a person-centred approach to care, articulated through the use of the nursing process as a work method, she was more likely to create the infrastructure which allowed the production and reproduction of emotional labour.

The sister's personal work preferences and priorities were more important in shaping the content of the nurses' work and learning than the medical labels of the wards (cf. Fretwell, 1982). The sister's emotional style of management was the key to the well-being of patients and nurses. Further research is required to identify the sources of her support which enabled her to make emotional labour an explicit part of her work.

Many of the issues explored in previous chapters are drawn together in Chapter 6 in order to further the understanding of emotional labour as a concept and its organisation in the hospital ward. Here I was particularly interested in how nurses in hospitals managed the ultimate emotional labour in caring for people who were dying, given that a majority go there to die. But as Field (1989) points out, busy hospital wards are not necessarily the most suitable place to die, and many people would prefer to stay at home but for the inadequacy of the community services. I found, as with other situations in which emotional labour was called for, that the ward sister's role was fundamental in putting death, dying and bereavement on the ward agenda. I also found that because students' feelings were rarely acknowledged in the open arena of the ward nor adequately addressed within their formal training they developed distancing strategies to keep them from involvement. They were unwilling to accept that they could be formally taught to 'react', preferring to see their learning about death and dying as experiential.

The penultimate chapter describes the students' caring trajectories and looks at the factors that shape their emotional careers. Students describe trajectories where they begin fresh and enthusiastic with an 'uncanny way' of getting to know their patients, but arrive at the end of three years' training 'cynical and disillusioned'. A number of caring factors were identified which influenced students' caring styles and capacity over time and their choice of future forms of emotional labour. Personal support was *ad hoc* throughout training, and personal relationships were fragmented between nurses and nurses and patients aggravated by the shift and allocation systems. I speculate that if students' individuality and caring commitment is repressed too often and for too long then it is likely that they will choose

141

hierarchical relations, stereotyping and labelling as preferred forms of emotional labour.

Melia (1984, 1987) noted the discontinuity suffered by student nurses, concluding that because of this they could not be regarded as following a true apprenticeship. Their rapid movement from ward to ward and shift to shift, as I found, militated against them working with the same nurse (trained or untrained) for any length of time.

Much attention has been given to this problem by members of the Project 2000 working groups. Students are likely to be allocated to fewer clinical areas and for longer periods. They will be supernumerary and require close supervision and support. The English National Board (1987), for example, suggests that 'each student must have a named supervisor or mentor in each practical placement'. On the basis of my findings I support this recommendation in principle, in that students will have a clearly identified person responsible for their teaching and assessment in each clinical allocation. However, there are a number of comments I would like to make. Firstly, whether this person is called a supervisor or a mentor is an issue. As we saw in this study, students felt uncomfortable with the idea of being 'supervised' in the sense of being 'checked every inch of the way'. But they also valued and requested more systematic support. If they are being 'supervised' in the psychiatric nursing or social work sense they will potentially receive this support and gain insights from their supervisor. Mentors also support and give insights to their mentees. But whether supervisor or mentor, this can only be done by forming a good relationship with the student. Given the importance of the nursing hierarchy in shaping relationships, and their fragmentary and discontinuous nature, three important recommendations emerge from my study. One is that the student nurse should be able to choose her supervisor/mentor; secondly this person should not be hierarchically threatening to her; and thirdly they should be able to continue their relationship throughout the student's training.

The duties of the mentor go far beyond those of the supervisor as teacher and assessor. The mentor must encourage and help shape the career of her student. She must be caring and able to offer advice and direction in the face of problems. She must also be an acknowledged expert in her own right (Bracken and Davies, 1989). Thus the mentor would make intelligible the student's learning experiences and provide her with a support

142

system that both enabled her to recognise and undertake emotional labour in a positive way.

In the NHS at the present time, the most likely people to supervise the students are either senior student nurses (as I found in my study) or recently qualified staff nurses. The staff nurses are prepared for their role by post-basic teaching and assessing courses validated by the national training boards. As yet there are not enough of them either to take on these roles or with the necessary personal and professional experience to do them well.

The UKCC is aware that measures must be taken to help trained nurses to meet the challenges generated by changes in education and practice. Proposals developed by the Post-Registration Education and Practice Project (PREPP) have recently been publicised (UKCC, 1990). The project recommends ways of keeping practioners up to date and preparing newly registered nurses to take on their new responsibilities. Like the mentor scheme for students, newly qualified nurses should have a period of support from designated 'preceptors'. These preceptors should be sufficently experienced to 'act as a role model' and 'evolve individual and learning methods in a flexible relationship'.

These recommendations suggest that emotional care and communication and encounter as part of nursing is being extended beyond the nurse–patient relationship to the working relationships between all levels of nurses. The call for nurses to undertake emotional labour, not only for patients, but also for colleagues, is growing. The UKCC believes that the 'health of the nation' depends on 'well-prepared and skilled' practitioners. But as my research shows, central to that relationship is an understanding of the emotional complexity of care.

The effects of emotional care on patient outcomes

To conclude, I will give the final words to the patients. One reason for doing this is to address the question that will be on the lips of general managers looking for cost-effectiveness and efficency. What effect does emotional labour have on patient outcomes? Positive forms of emotional labour certainly make them feel better. And there is sufficient evidence that negative forms of emotional labour which stereotype and label patients can be positively harmful. Some years ago there was a television docu-drama which caused a great stir amongst the public and hospital world alike. It was called 'Major Implications' (MacMillan, 1980). It was about a woman who was admitted to hospital for minor surgery and ended up having a large proportion of her bowel removed. What happened was the following. The woman, a successful middle-class artist, divorced with two children with a new partner, decided to have a sterilisation. It became clear from the beginning that the nurses did not approve of her decision. They were coldly polite to her. On return from surgery she did not recover as quickly as was expected. On the first postoperative day she was encouraged, according to the routine, to get up and wash herself. The nurses dismissed her complaints of nausea and were not even sympathetic when she fainted. Because they did not approve of her and resented her middle-class articulateness they labelled her as a 'difficult patient'. Consequently they failed to take her complaints seriously. The doctors reacted similarly and there was collusion between them and the nurses. Eventually, after five days of decline, culminating in the frank symptoms of intestinal obstruction, the unfortunate woman was rushed to the operating theatre. Part of her bowel had to be excised and she was left with a permanent colostomy and a ruined life. If the nurses had looked beyond the stereotype they might have saved her physical and emotional suffering.

But when nurses engage in positive emotional labour their effects on their patients are profound, as the following account, by a patient, demonstrates.

P. When I discovered my diagnosis, I wanted to share it or get rid of it if you like. If I try to hide things then that just makes matters worse.

Q. Do you feel you've had permission to do that . . . ?

P. Yes. The nurses have been brilliant. They're such good listeners. They've held my hand literally and metaphorically. They've said exactly the right things at the right time. I've never been patronised by either the doctors or nurses. If I felt they were hiding something that would make me worry and effect me emotionally and probably physically as well. After I'd been here a few days the nurses must have guessed that I needed to talk. They'd obviously read my notes. One nurse came to me and we held hands, it was a real comfort. It's difficult to describe but there was no fear. It was so natural and it had a calming influence even though I cried. It happened on two different occasions. But to give yourself a chance physically you need to have the emotional side there helping you.

The patient makes clear links between the emotional and physical aspects of her care. She describes caring gestures, the little things that make her feel qualitatively different: nurses who recognised she needed to talk, were good listeners, held her hand, took away her fear and had a calming influence on her. She described them as 'brilliant' indicating that she recognised they had skills, but also implied that these caring gestures were 'natural', both in the sense of intuitive and genuine. Emotional labour does make a difference and care matters to patients, but it is still in danger of being marginalised.

The skill lies in the nurse who is able to recognise that emotional labour is needed and may be required in different forms for different patients. Not everyone wants to hold hands and show their tears in front of others. Would the emotional labour have taken a different form if the genders of the actors were reversed or their class, race and cultures were different? Did the patient make a better recovery from surgery than if she hadn't been emotionally supported in this way? Had the nurses been formally taught to listen and recognise the patient's need to talk? How did they feel after their encounter and who supported them and gave them feedback?

There is clearly scope for much more research in the area of emotion and health care. The pressure is clearly on to intensify nursing work through changes in nurses' education, work organisation and NHS managers looking to their budgets. Nurses are at the front line of care and they do make a difference. This book has shown some of the ways how and why.

Methodological appendix

The material presented in this book is loosely based on doctoral research. The aim of the research was to study the relationship between the quality of nursing and the ward as a learning environment for student nurses. I used a variety of research methods and tools in the study (Smith, 1987). My main finding was that the relationship between quality of nursing and ward learning is articulated through the sister's emotional style of management. In the book I concentrate on the nature of the relationship and the emotional components of care and learning to care.

In this appendix I describe only those methods I used to re-experience the world of the student nurse and construct their training trajectories. My key research perspectives were participant observation, grounded theory and feminist sociology. I chose qualitative sociological methods because of their flexibility for data handling, hypothesis formulation and exploration of complex social phenomena.

Participant observation

The classification of the participant observer role is well documented in the literature (Gold, 1969; Denzin, 1970; Pearsall, 1970). The complete participant role is theoretically inspired by qualitative, interpretivist research traditions, whereas the complete observer role tends towards positivism and quantification common in the natural and medical sciences. Collins (1984) proposes an alternative classification in which he describes the complete observer role as 'unobtrusive observation' and the complete participant as 'participant comprehension' in which the act of participating is central and essential to the method. The researcher enters the research setting seeking to maximise rather than minimise her interaction so as to grow both in competence and comprehension of the 'native culture'. I aimed to emulate this approach during participant observation on the wards. In the classroom I was a complete observer during the lectures, but in the breaks I interacted with the students and teachers as an active participant.

I adopted Melia's application of the participant observer role during interview with students and their teachers. Melia (1982) contends that 'the close involvement of the researcher in the production of the data is as true of the informal interview method of data production as it is of participant observation' (p. 329). Not only was Melia familiar with the social setting from which her subjects originated, but she used the interview as a forum through which to interact with them in the production of data.

Grounded theory

Grounded theory is an integrated, qualitative research approach promoted by Glaser and Strauss (1967). They describe how grounded theory can be used for the gathering, handling and analysis of data in order to generate 'modes of conceptualisation for describing and explaining'. Glaser and Strauss emphasise that the aim of their research approach is to generate rather than to verify theory through 'theoretical sampling'. Theoretical sampling is described as the joint collection, coding and analysis of data whereby the researcher decides what further data to collect and where to find them based on data already collected, coded and analysed. Thus, theory is seen as 'a process and ever developing entity' through the creation of conceptual categories and their properties and hypotheses or general relations among them.

Feminist sociology

The development of feminist sociology has made a significant contribution to both sociological and nursing research. Bell and Roberts (1984) draw attention to the emergence of a 'strong programme' of feminist sociology since the late 1970s. Feminist sociology is concerned not only with raising gender issues in the

147

formulation of research problems, methods and analysis, but also takes account of the 'differences in the way that research is organised, carried out and written up as being based on the gender of the researcher' (Bell and Roberts, 1984, p. 3).

Oakley (1981) challenges conventional 'male paradigms' which mystify 'the researcher and the researched as objective instruments of data production' and condemn 'personal involvement' as 'dangerous bias' (p. 58). Oakley sees the use of subjectivity as essential to both the interviewing process and production of data.

Indeed, feminist researchers highlight the vulnerability of research subjects especially during interview, in which traditionally the researcher 'takes' all the information on offer without reciprocity or responsibility (Stanley and Wise, 1983). These observations are particularly relevant to the study of nursing since nurses are especially vulnerable to external authority structures. The researcher has a responsibility to protect the vulnerability of persons under study. James, for example, periodically made outrageous statements to remind people that there was a researcher in their midst (James, 1984).

Webb (1984b) has explicitly put feminist sociology on the nursing research agenda. Drawing on the writings of feminist sociologists she describes feminist research 'as critique' which:

aims specifically to work towards defining alternatives and understanding everyday experience in order to bring about change. Analysis and critique of research methods leads on to analysis and critique in the research context through consciousness raising both for researcher and researched. (p. 250)

The contribution of feminist perspectives to nursing research is particularly pertinent, given that it is a predominantly female occupation and nurses are involved in traditionally female roles and work activities prescribed by the predominantly male medical profession. Feminist research can be seen to value yet develop qualitative research traditions by making gender relations visible at the level of both researcher and researched.

Organisation of the research

The study was organised in four phases. For clarity, they are categorised and described as if they were distinct and took place

148

sequentially. However, in practice, there was some degree of overlap between each phase.

Phase one: January – June of Year I

Exploratory work on a variety of hospital wards. Three months were spent on one medical ward participating and observing the practice and learning of nursing. A variety of research tools and methods were tried out in order to explore ways of conceptualising the variables (quality of nursing and the ward learning environment) and to select appropriate techniques, settings and subjects for describing and explaining their interrelationship.

Phase two: April of Year I – June of Year II

The school of nursing. During the first few weeks of this phase of the research, volunteer groups of students were interviewed and discussion groups held to identify topics to be addressed during interview. Teachers were also interviewed. The Fretwell rating questionnaire on the ward learning environment was tried out with four groups of students at different stages of training. All the students were undertaking medical nursing on their first or third ward (first-years) and at the beginning or end of their third year. Preliminary analysis of questionnaire data yielded valuable findings, and confirmed the usefulness of the instrument as a measure of students' perceptions of the ward learning environment. It was decided therefore to continue using the questionnaire as a method of data collection.

Classes were observed and decisions made about which ones to select to observe in depth. The content of timetables for the medical modules was recorded and analysed. A first- and third-year group of students were selected for observation (sets A and B respectively) and a random sample from each was recruited for interview.

Phase three: November of Year I – June of Year II

Three in-depth study periods on selected medical wards of eight weeks, during which the researcher participated in and observed the practice and learning of nursing using instruments and methods from the exploratory phase of the study.

149

Phase four: July of Year II – July of Year IV

In-depth analysis and writing up.

Details of subjects studied

Details of the subjects studied are given, according to the research techniques for which they were recruited.

Questionnaires on the ward learning environment

524 rating questionnaires were completed by 392 learners from 19 sets, with respect to 12 medical wards, i.e. 132 learners completed the questionnaire twice during their week in school following their allocation. In all, questionnaires were completed by a total of 188 first-year students and 204 third-year students. Response rates in the first year and junior third years were almost 100 per cent. The non-response rate for senior third-years was 25 per cent. One reason for the drop in response rates at the end of training was that classroom sessions were no longer compulsory.

The majority of the respondents were female, representing the composition of the students at City. The maximum number of male students who could have filled in the questionnaire at least once was 10.

The data yielded from the open-ended questions at the end of the questionnaire (questions 37–41) were based on the stratified random sampling of students' comments. A baseline of 10 comments per ward from students at each stage of training was sought. A total of 79 respondents were selected, which yielded approximately 20 replies from each group.

Interviews

The student sample comprised 18 volunteers, 8 students who had been approached by me, and 15 students who had been randomly selected from the first and third year of training.

In summary a total of 16 first-year students were interviewed, in groups, in pairs or individually. Four students were interviewed three times, one twice and eleven once. The interviews were conducted during modules 1, 3 and 4. Four students in the random sample from set A were involved in one discussion group. In addition, a total of 12 students (two of whom were also interviewed) from another set took part in three group discussions during their first-year medical ward allocation.

A total of 15 third-years were interviewed. Ten were interviewed once and five three times. Ten interviews were conducted at the beginning and end of module 12 and 15 during module 15 at the end of training.

The majority of the students were women. There were only four male students in the population from which the sample was drawn, one of whom was selected. The age range of the group was 18–24 for first-years and 20–28 for third-years.

Details of parents' occupations were not available for all students, but they included a number of fathers who were doctors, an accountant, a managing director, a press officer and a print worker. A number of mothers were nurses. All students were British, and only one was non-white.

All the students had the minimal educational qualifications for entry to the City school of nursing of five O levels and at least one A level pass. Four of the students were also university graduates.

The sisters on all four study wards agreed to be interviewed. Their ages ranged from 28–38 years. One of them had been in her post for three years, two for four years, and one for ten years. Three out of the four sisters had undertaken post-basic nurse education in intensive care nursing. One had a degree and two had trained at the City Hospital. The two other sisters had also trained in London teaching hospitals.

In total, five tutors from year 1 were interviewed and four tutors from Year 3. One clinical teacher was interviewed. One psychiatric tutor was interviewed. Thus, a total of eleven nurse teachers were interviewed. Three had degrees, two had trained at City Hospital and all had undertaken post-basic nurse education in addition to nurse teacher training. Their ages ranged from 30–50 years.

The biographical details of the patients are given according to the wards on which they were interviewed and from where they were discharged. On Kinder ward, only three patients were interviewed. All were male. Two were over 75 and the other interviewee was 36. Ten patients were interviewed on Ronda ward. All were female. Their ages ranged from 41–81. On Windermere ward, eight patients were interviewed. Seven were men and one a woman. Their ages ranged from 26–86. On Edale ward, ten female patients were interviewed. Their ages ranged from 30–85.

In summary, a total of 31 patients were interviewed. They could be characterised as white, lower middle- and middle-class, based on their occupations. A number of the older respondents were retired. Only two of the respondents were non-British. Their length of hospitalisation varied from two days to eight weeks and they suffered from a variety of acute and chronic conditions. Some patients were suffering from life-threatening conditions such as lymphoma and advanced coronary artery disease. Others were at the beginning of their illness trajectory and had been admitted for investigations.

Non-participant observation in the school of nursing

During non-participant observation in the school of set A's Foundation Unit, modules 1 and 3, a total of 26 from a potential 238 sessions were observed. A total of six nurse tutors were observed. The majority of them were Year 1 tutors.

Examination of biographical information for the first-year students yields the following data: 20 students in the group, including one male student, with an average of eight O level and 1.8 A level subjects passed. Their ages ranged from 18–22. By module 3, three students had left.

Non-participant observation in the school for the third-year group included 39 sessions out of a potential 124. A total of five different nurse teachers were observed. The majority of them were Year 3 tutors.

Examination of biographical information for the third-years yields the following data: a total of 29 students, including three male students, with an average of 7.5 O levels and 1.7 A levels. They included two graduates. The students had an age range of 20–28 years, and were generally regarded as having an above average age range for a group of student nurses; the majority of the set were not direct entrants to nursing from secondary school. They were therefore not regarded as a representative group of students for City school of nursing, most of whom had come directly from secondary school to start training.

152

Observer participation

On each of the four study wards, the ward establishment of trained staff in addition to the sister varied from eight staff nurses on Edale ward to six on Windermere ward and five each on Kinder and Ronda wards.

Each ward had an average allocation of 10 student nurses during their first- and third-year medical placements. Numbers varied in each module according to size of the set, from zero in some instances to three in others. In an eight-week observation period, I would expect to have contact with an average of 17 nurses at different stages of training.

A number of students featured in all data sets described above, i.e. survey interviewing; document analysis; direct observation and observer participation. Others appeared in one to three of the sets. The choice of techniques, settings and subjects permitted the students as the principal actors to be well represented in the study.

Methods of data collection

I applied the notion of 'triangulation' or a multi-method research approach to my study (Denzin, 1970). These methods are described in the following sub-sections.

Ward learning environment rating questionnaire

Fretwell's questionnaire on the ward learning environment was given to students at the end of their medical ward allocation (Fretwell, 1985).

Thirty-six items were grouped in six sections, A, B, C, D, E and F. Each section looked at different characteristics of the ward learning environment. Section A contained seven items which asked respondents to rate the ward learning environment in terms of workload, staffing levels and mix (items 4, 6 and 7). Items 1, 3 and 5 rated the respondent's perception of potential and actual learning on the ward. Item 2 rated the extent to which students felt happy with their ward experience. As such it could be seen as an indicator of their general feeling of well-being whilst on the ward.

153

Section B rated 'Ward Atmosphere/Staff Relations' on seven items. Section C rated 'Ward Teaching' on ten items. Section D rated 'Provision of Learning Opportunities' on six items. Section E related to 'Patient Care' and contained five items.

Responses to each statement on items 1–35 were on a five-point Likert scale from 'strongly agree' (5) to 'strongly disagree' (1). Section F, on 'Anxiety and Stress', asked students to tick whether they experienced anxiety or stress: 'Frequently', 'Occasionally', 'Not very often', or 'Never' whilst working on the ward. Students were awarded a score according to the frequency with which they experienced stress or anxiety from 3 (Frequently) to 0 (Never).

There were also five open-ended questions at the end of the questionnaire which asked students for general comments on ward learning. They included questions on causes of stress or anxiety; identification of most valuable and least valuable educational experiences; suggestions for improving teaching and learning and an opportunity to make any additional comments about the ward.

The questionnaire was self-administered and had been tested for reliability and validity. In terms of validity of the questionnaire, Fretwell (1985) argued that it had 'content validity' because it was based on previous research findings (Fretwell, 1982). Items on the questionnaire which were said to be indicators of a 'good' learning environment were validated by other researchers (Orton, 1981; Ogier, 1982). Fretwell also found that comments made in questionnaires and during informal conversation with trained and student nurses confirmed its validity as a tool for evaluating the ward learning environment. Fretwell ran a number of reliability tests on the questionnaire, and on a shortened version of it, which was used in the present study (reported in Fretwell, 1985).

Semi-structured interviews with sisters and patients

The ward sister interview schedule was organised around questions rather than topics and aimed at finding out about the ward sister's resources and how she organised nursing on 'a typical day', allocated the work, and received feedback on what had been done (Pembrey, 1980). These questions gave insights into the ward sister's interpretation of the nursing process and supervision of students. Additional topics included student

154

nurse teaching and learning; role of and contact with the school of nursing; and nature of the work and the learning material on the ward.

Coser's (1962) patient interview guide was used to explore patients' perceptions of quality of nursing. Patients were asked to describe their 'ideal' doctor, nurse or patient; also their experience of hospitalisation from the point of view of resources and contact with personnel. Communication and interpersonal skills and the role of student nurses as care givers emerged as important topics for further discussion.

Observer participation: participant observation on four wards and interviews with students and teachers

The student nurse interview agenda was organised around the following topics: general overview of training; integration of classroom teaching and ward practice; teaching and learning: identification of key people and incidents; the wards: nature of the work and quality of nursing; formal training requirements; and the role of the school of nursing. A similar agenda was used during student discussion groups.

The nurse tutor interview agenda was organised around the following topics: background prior to and reasons for becoming a nurse teacher; the school–ward contact; theoretical content of training; student nurses' personal and learning needs; and the role of the school of nursing.

The nursing process, patterns of ward allocation and the teaching and learning of interpersonal skills and communication were added to the schedule of topics for both students and teachers as the research progressed.

Direct observation
Non-participant observation of selected classes in the school of nursing

The field notes from participant observation on the wards and non-participant observation in the classroom were analysed concurrently with data collection as were the content of the plan of training and medical module timetables. The findings thus obtained were used as evidence to illustrate emergent concepts.

155

Document analysis

Student biographical data, plan of student nurse training, timetables, prospectus, school progress reports and national recruitment campaign literature.

Data analysis

The ward learning environment questionnaires were prepared for computer analysis. A random sample of open-ended comments was analysed manually.

Fretwell's system of analysis was used. A mean score was calculated for each item by allotting scores of 5, 4, 3, 2, 1 for most to least favourable responses. A mean score for each section (A, B, C, D, E) was derived from the sum of individual item scores for that section. Overall mean scores were also calculated. These scores represented the mean of the sum of item scores 1–35. Wards were ranked on the basis of these scores.

An anxiety and stress rating for each ward was obtained by calculating a mean score from the number of times that students allotted scores of 3, 2, 1 or 0 for the frequency with which they experienced these emotions on the ward. The rating was from 3.0 (frequently experienced) to 0 (never experienced). It is possible that students had difficulties in distinguishing between the intermediate categories of 'occasionally' experienced and 'not very often'. In retrospect it might have been more appropriate to re-classify the categories as 'sometimes' and 'seldom'.

The overall ward ratings represented the students' perceptions of a ward's overall rating as a learning environment. Section scores B, C, D and E represented a measure of the students' perception of the ward atmosphere/staff relations. Scores C and D are measures of the students' perceptions of ward teaching and the provision of learning opportunities, respectively. Item score 36 is an indicator of students' perception of stress or anxiety experienced on a ward.

Items 1–7 contained in section A of the questionnaire do not form an index of a discrete dimension of the ward learning environment. Rather they are related to individual items associated with their perceptions of the ward learning environment, such as feelings of happiness, staffing levels, workload, potential and actual learning.

Glaser and Strauss (1967) illustrate the potential overlap between qualitative and quantitative data analysis which I applied to the analysis of the Fretwell questionnaires. Thus data may be collected using a quantitative instrument but analysed in a qualitative way. For example, single items and/or indices of concepts on a questionnaire may in their view be used in bivariate analysis. In this way, 'general relationships between the items and/or indices are established which suggest hypotheses for an emerging theory' (p. 190). Glaser and Strauss suggest that if relationships between variables consistently appear and can be integrated into a coherent theory, then the items and indices achieve their own validation. As with data obtained using qualitative methods, researchers are urged to be flexible in the way they handle it to 'maintain a sensitivity to all possible theoretical relevances' (p. 194).

Thus, theoretical rather than statistical sampling guided the analysis of quantitative as well as qualitative data collecting instruments and techniques. Two variable relationships were sought from the item and section questionnaire scores. The theoretical ordering and interaction between variables were suggested by the qualitative data analysis.

Applying these principles, item and section scores were selected from the Fretwell questionnaires for bivariate analysis which had theoretical relevance to the research question under study and to confirm working hypotheses. Differences between wards and stage of training according to module were also examined.

Statistical methods

Comparisons of mean scores derived from the Fretwell questionnaire between pairs of wards were conducted using Gabriel's test. This is a multiple comparison procedure for unequal sized groups similar to Tukey's range test for equal sized groups (Kendall and Stuart, 1968).

Relationships between the scores on different scales across the 12 wards were tested using Pearson's correlation coefficient. As the mean score for each ward was the sum of many observations, it was possible to treat these means as continuous.

Since for the testing of the null hypothesis of no relationship only one variable need be normal and the test is fairly robust, the data were well suited to this method.

In addition, a random sample of students' responses to the open-ended questions at the end of the questionnaire was also analysed for consistent themes. These themes were used to form categories. Comments were then classified under the appropriate categories. For example, replies to question 37 on causes of stress and anxiety were classified under the following categories: nature of the work; staffing levels; staff relations; and feelings about self/work/staff relations. Replies to question 38 on work and other experiences valuable to learning were classified under the following categories: nature of the work according to patient characteristics; basic, technical and affective nursing required (Goddard, 1953); specialist medical knowledge, investigations and treatment; formal teaching; staff relations; and effects on feelings. The inferences drawn from the replies to the open-ended questions on the questionnaire are tentative, since, with the exception of question 38, they are based on a small number of replies. The comments are used to complement data obtained from the rating sections of the questionnaire, interviews and field observations.

Data yielded from the interviews and fieldwork observation were analysed as the research progressed in order to decide what further data to collect and where to find them in future fieldwork.

Analysis took place using theoretical sampling described above. Analysis was also comparative in that data collected from a variety of settings (wards, classroom) and groups (students, ward sisters, tutors, patients) were used to check out whether original evidence was correct. As Glaser and Strauss observe: 'Facts are replicated with comparative evidence either internally (within a study) or externally (outside) or both'.

But for Glaser and Strauss the main goal of comparative analysis is to generate two kinds of theory defined as 'substantive' and 'formal'. They define substantive theory in the following way: 'that developed for a substantive, or empirical area of sociological inquiry', e.g. patient care, professional education. Formal theory is defined as that 'developed for a formal or conceptual area of sociological inquiry', e.g. socialisation, authority and power.

Substantive theory must precede formal theory, otherwise 'the consequence is often a forcing of data, as well as a neglect of relevant concepts and hypotheses that may emerge' (p. 34). Thus:

The constant comparing of many groups draws the sociologist's attention to their many similarities and differences. Considering these leads him to generate abstract categories and their properties which since they emerge from the data, will clearly be important to a theory explaining the kind of behaviour under observation. (Glaser and Strauss 1967, p. 36)

It is suggested that, in order to avoid contamination of data at this early stage, the researcher should 'ignore' the existing literature relevant to the research problem. Bulmer (1983) notes the difficulty of doing this in order 'to keep one's mind altogether free from presuppositions or prior conceptualisations' in areas that have been well researched. Thus, in my study it was impossible to 'ignore' those areas of the literature which had been well researched and were of relevance to the research problem, such as ward learning.

Throughout the data collection and analysis the literature was regularly reviewed and used as Glaser and Strauss suggested to ascertain if any existing formal theories might aid in the generation of substantive theories from the emergent conceptual categorisations and propositions. In the present study the definition and analysis of 'emotional labour' (Hochschild, 1983), was identified and used in this way.

The validity and reliability of the data obtained using qualitative strategies are an integral part of an approach such as grounded theory, which seeks to generate, rather than verify, theory from the data. Thus validity is implicit when data are simultaneously collected, handled and analysed to shape ongoing data collection and to develop and confirm working hypotheses. Similarly, reliability is ascertained during the participant observer role in that the researcher, over time and with increasing familiarity, is able to check the accuracy and recurrence of the data in a number of settings and from a number of participants.

Patients' interview guide (Coser, 1962)

1. When you are sick, would you rather be at home or in hospital?
2. What do you miss most while you are in the hospital?
3. What is your idea of a good doctor?
4. What is your idea of a good nurse?
5. What is your idea of a good patient?
6. How do you like the rounds?
7. How do you like the wards?
8. Are there any suggestions that you would care to make for a possible improvement of the patients' comfort?
9. Are you ever bored or restless while you are in the hospital?
10. What will be the first thing you will do when you get home?

PRIVATE AND CONFIDENTIAL

WARD LEARNING ENVIRONMENT RATING QUESTIONNAIRE

Ward . . . .

Student ☐   Pupil ☐   Trained Nurse ☐

(Please tick)

The following statements are concerned with nurse training in the ward. For each statement please indicate your opinion by placing a tick (√) in one of the five boxes. There are no right or wrong answers, but please try to avoid the 'uncertain' column unless you really cannot agree or disagree. If you wish to clarify or explain your choice, make your comments in the box provided.

Note: The term 'learner' is intended to include both student and pupil nurses.
'Sister' applies to charge nurses.

SECTION A (Questions 1 to 3 to be answered by student and pupil nurses only)	Strongly Agree	Agree	Uncertain	Disagree	Strongly Disagree	Comments
1. This was a good ward for student/ pupil learning.						
2. I am happy with the experience I have had on this ward.						
3. I learnt very much on this ward.						
(Remaining questions to be answered by everyone)						
4. The number of staff is adequate for the workload.						
5. There is very much to learn on this ward.						
6. There are enough trained nurses in relation to learners and auxiliaries.						
7. The workload does not interfere with teaching or learning.						

1982 REVISION Copyright: Dr Joan Fretwell, Department of Sociology,
University of Warwick, Coventry.

and: – West Midlands Regional Health Authority.

1984: Permission given to P A Smith to use the questionnaire.

162

SECTION B. WARD ATMOSPHERE/STAFF RELATIONS On this ward, the sister and trained nurses:-	Strongly Agree	Agree	Uncertain	Disagree	Strongly Disagree	Comments
8. Provide an atmosphere which is good to work in.						
9. Are concerned about what a student is thinking or feeling.						
10. Are available and approachable.						
11. Give reprimands in private.						
12. Praise and encourage the learner in her work.						
13. Work as a team with learners.						
14. Keep staff and learners well informed about ward activities.						
SECTION C. WARD TEACHING						
15. Sister devotes a lot of her time to teaching learners.						
16. Trained nurses on the ward teach regularly.						
17. Clinical teachers teach regularly on the ward.						
18. Consultants are interested in teaching.						
19. There are regular sessions, in which trained nurses discuss the nursing care of patients.						
20. The ward report is used as an occasion for teaching learners.						
21. Trained nurses teach as they work with learners.						
22. Sister initiates teaching.						
23. Learning objectives are in use on this ward.						
24. Sister accords teaching and learning activities a place in the routine.						

SECTION D. PROVISION OF LEARNING OPPORTUNITIES	Strongly Agree	Agree	Uncertain	Disagree	Strongly Disagree	Comments
25. Trained and learner nurses work together giving a full range of care, e.g. bathing and dressing.						
26. Sister and trained nurses give learners an opportunity to watch or perform new procedures.						
27. Sister attaches great importance to the learning needs of student and pupil nurses.						
28. Sister gives learners the opportunity to read case notes and text books.						
29. Learners are given an opportunity to use their initiative and discretion.						
30. Learners are taught on doctors' rounds.						
SECTION E. PATIENT CARE						
31. Sister promotes good staff/ patient relationships.						
32. Patients receive the best attention and nursing care.						
33. Patients get plenty of opportunity to discuss their feelings and anxieties.						
34. Nursing care is tailored to meet the individual needs of patients.						
35. Patient allocation rather than task allocation is the practice on this ward.						

SECTION F. ANXIETY AND STRESS

36. Do/did you experience anxiety or stress whilst working on this ward?

        Frequently ☐   Occasionally ☐   Not very often ☐   Never ☐

        (Please tick)

37. Identify the main cause(s) of any stress or anxiety on this ward.

38. What work and other experiences on this ward were most valuable for your education?

39. What work and other experiences were least valuable for your education?

40. Have you any suggestions for improving teaching and learning on this ward? If so please give details.

41. In case you have any other comments to make about the ward, would you write them below

THANK YOU FOR YOUR CO-OPERATION

Appendix A: City school of nursing plan of training

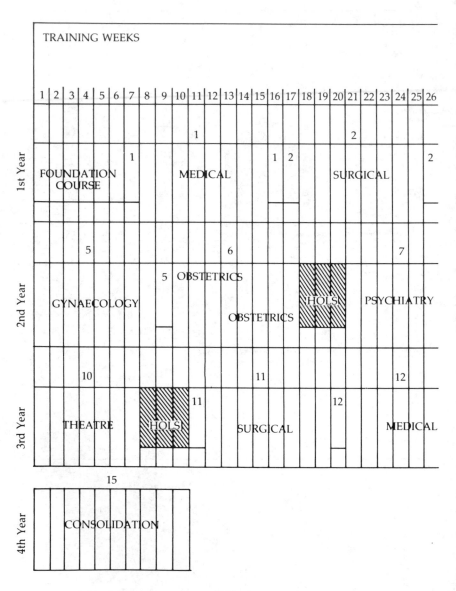

27	28	29	30	31	32	33	34	35	36	37	38	39	40	41	42	43	44	45	46	47	48	49	50	51	52

| | | | | | 3 | | | | | | | | | 4 | | | | | | | | | | | |
| HOLS | 3 | | | MEDICAL | | | | | | | 3 | 4 | | SURGICAL | | | | | | 4 | HOLS | 5 |

| | | | | | 8 | | | | | | | | | 9 | | | | | | | | | | | |
| 8 | | | PAEDIATRICS | | | | | | | 8 | HOLS | 9 | | GERIATRICS | | | | | | 9 | |

| | | | | | 13 | | | | | | | | | 14 | | | | | | | | | | | |
| 13 | | | ACCIDENT/ EMERGENCY | | | | | | | HOLS | 14 | | MEDICAL | | | | | | 15 | |

167

Appendix B: Student nurse assessment form

(The form which follows on pp. 168–74 is based on King's Fund/GNC Working Party recommendations. See also *Assessment. A guide for the completion of progress reports on nurses in training* (King Edward's Hospital Fund for London, 1972).)

STUDENT NURSE PROGRESS ASSESSMENT FORM

PRELIMINARY INTERVIEW

Date

Note special tuition requested by student, and any comments made on particular weaknesses and difficulties: it may also be helpful to note any omissions revealed in record of practical instruction.

Signature

FINAL INTERVIEW   Date

1. Any further comments by assessor

2. OVERALL GRADING: Review your assessments and decide appropriate overall grading (tick in box)

outstandingly good	very good	good-satisfactory	just good enough	not good enough

Signature   Post held

WHEN YOU COMPLETE THIS FORM

Try to remember that you are assessing a student over a PERIOD OF TIME. It is all too easy to allow particular incidents to influence both your assessment of a particular quality and also your general impression of overall merit.

Under each item in turn put a tick in the box which best fits the nurse's usual performance. If you cannot assess an individual on any particular item, write N/A for 'not applicable', and give your reasons under 'Comments'.

Do not hesitate to give X (very high) or Y (low) gradings where deserved. Try not to let the nurse's strength or weakness in one quality cloud your judgement of her/his standing in another. Praise should be given where it is deserved.

It is quite normal for an individual to be above average in some respects and to fall short in others.

Comments are always helpful particularly to explain an unusual grading or when an unqualified tick might not present a true picture.

X

Y

I. APPLICATION TO WORK

I. APPLICATION TO WORK	X applies	Tendency to X	Average	Tendency to Y	Y applies	
1. Exceptionally industrious; a very keen and willing worker.						Does little more than she/he has to; appears half-hearted and indifferent.
2. More active than most in using opportunities to extend knowledge and skill.						Shows little active interest in using opportunities to increase knowledge and skill.
3. Outstandingly quick in grasping essentials.						Sometimes has difficulty in grasping essentials.
4. Always punctual in arriving for duty.						Not always punctual in arriving for duty.
5. Consistently prompt in carrying out duties. Timing excellent.						Does not yet keep to time very well; tends to hold up work.

COMMENTS:

II. QUALITY OF WORK	X applies	Tendency to X	Average	Tendency to Y	Y applies	
6. Maintains a very high standard when carrying out nursing procedures.						Does not show a good enough standard in carrying out nursing procedures.

#			Rating			
7.	Makes excellent application of theoretical knowledge to practical work.					Often appears not to apply her/his theoretical knowledge to the practical situation.
8.	Work shows a consistently high standard of attention to detail and finish.					Work does not always show sufficient attention to detail and finish.
9.	Invariably carries out instructions reliably without supervision.					Needs more supervision than most; cannot always be relied upon to carry out instructions completely.
10.	Unusually observant. Always reports signs, symptoms and other relevant information.					Not yet sufficiently observant; sometimes omits to observe/pass on/relevant information.
11.	(a) Exceptionally self-reliant and resourceful. (b) Shows excellent ability to plan and complete own work/organise work of others.					(a) Needs more than the usual amount of support to cope with routine work. (b) Has not yet learnt to organize/own work effectively/work of others.
12.	Can always be relied upon to record promptly all necessary clinical data.					Inclined to be dilatory in recording necessary clinical data.
13.	Regularly produces excellent reports and records, well written, complete and clearly expressed.					Written reports and records are not always complete and clear; more practice needed.

COMMENTS:

171

X
                      Y

III. ATTITUDE TO PATIENTS	X applies	Tendency to X	Average	Tendency to Y	Y applies	
14. Successfully anticipates and meets the physical needs of patients.						Sometimes fails to recognise and meet patients' physical needs.
15. Shows exceptional understanding of patients as individual persons.						Seldom manages to adapt her/his approach to suit the needs of individuals.
16. Shows outstanding skill in gaining the confidence and co-operation of patients; tactful and considerate.						As yet unskilled in gaining the full confidence and co-operation of patients.
17. Shows better ability than most in dealing tactfully and courteously with patients' relatives and visitors.						Sometimes omits to show courtesy and understanding in dealing with patients' relatives and visitors.

COMMENTS:

172

IV. ATTITUDE TO CO-WORKERS	X applies	Tendency to X	Average	Tendency to Y	Y applies	
18. Very well accepted by nurse collea-gues; works well as member of a team.						Sometimes appears to have difficulties in working as a member of nursing team.
19. Gives alert and very efficient pro-fessional assistance to doctors in the clinical situation.						Apt to be casual in manner and insuffi-ciently informed when working with the medical staff.
20. Distinguished by courtesy and helpfulness towards other members of the hospital staff.						Sometimes appears rather off-hand in dealings with other members of the hospital staff.
21. Responds with good grace to instructions/advice. Makes the most of constructive criticism.						Often appears reluctant to accept instruction/advice/constructive criti-cism.
22. Highly successful in the instruc-tion and supervision of others.						Does not yet display much ability in instructing and supervising others.

COMMENTS:

V. PROFESSIONAL BEHAVIOUR	X applies	Tendency to X	Average	Tendency to Y	Y applies
23. Always very neat and well groomed – wears uniform correctly.					Not always neat and well groomed – uniform sometimes worn incorrectly.
24. (a) Demonstrates understanding of the need for quietness in speech and manner. (b) Protects patients from undue noise at all times.					(a) Appears unaware of the need for quietness in speech and manner. (b) Does little to control or reduce noise in the ward environment unless constantly reminded.
25. Notably poised and effective even in situations of stress.					Easily ruffled; is put out by unusual or difficult situations.

COMMENTS:

Appendix C: General course philosophy, aims and objectives

Note: The course philosophy, aims and objectives presented here, are taken from the General Nursing Council for England and Wales' Training Syllabus 1977. The City school curriculum papers were loosely based on this syllabus. I have not given details of the City programme to protect anonymity.

The Syllabus sets out in broad terms the subjects to be studied during training for Registration in the general part of the Register maintained by the General Nursing Council for England and Wales.

The concept underlying this syllabus is that of total patient care but for convenience the syllabus is divided into three main sections; nursing, the study of the individual and the nature and cause of disease together with its prevention and treatment. These three aspects of patient care should be learned concurrently throughout training. In this way the various needs of patients will be closely linked together; their needs as individuals and as patients requiring nursing and specialised care and rehabilitation.

The patient in hospital cannot be considered in isolation from the community and the nurse must be aware of the services provided by statutory authorities and voluntary organisations to help and safeguard individuals in their home and at work. The nurse also has an important part to play as a health teacher and must have a knowledge of the factors in the environment which give rise to ill-health since she will be called upon to advise patients and their relatives on how to care for themselves and their family in the way which will promote a state of physical and mental well-being.

Length of the course

The period of training is normally 156 weeks exclusive of excess sick leave and special leave.

Amount of teaching time

The total amount of time allocated for study blocks or study days during a 156 week training should not be less than 120 days (24 weeks). As programmes are developed which integrate theoretical and practical learning it is important to ensure that learning/teaching sessions within practical experiences are taken into account in the final record of "theoretical instruction". The length of the introductory course should be a minimum of 30 days (6 weeks) or a maximum of 40 days (8 weeks). It should provide a broad introduction and the opportunity to learn and practise basic nursing skills.

Examinations

Student nurses will be made aware of their progress as the course progresses and will be required to pass written and practical examinations prior to Registration.

PRACTICAL EXPERIENCES REQUIRED FOR THE TRAINING OF NURSES FOR ADMISSION TO THE GENERAL PART OF THE REGISTER

Definition of overall aims and learning objectives for the course

When defining the overall aims and the learning objectives for the course it will be important to identify the common core of the curriculum and the expected outcomes of the whole course: the synthesis of nursing knowledge, nursing skills and the body of beliefs and values which support a code of professional practice. The stages of the nursing process, as described by Professor Jean McFarlane, and others, is helpful in offering a theoretical framework for practice.

The use of this method commits all concerned in the various caring/learning situations to a shared approach and a common purpose.

176

Practical experiences

The majority of experiences will be gained in hospital, but steps should be taken to include some aspects of community care by arranging experience in community/home nursing preferably by incorporating suitable placements to enable the students to study home and hospital care in one or more periods of experience, e.g. during the study of the care of children or the care of the elderly. The aim should be to provide as a total, a minimum of 60 hours within a 3 year training, excluding any specific teaching sessions but including 'on-the-job' teaching.

In selecting the areas of inclusion and building these up into a curriculum it should be possible to ensure that student nurses have the opportunity to learn the following aspects of care:–

Initial care in illness: planned and emergency admission to hospital.
High and medium dependency care.
Preparation for self-care following discharge from hospital.
Continuing care for patients with long-term disability or recurrent illness necessitating re-admission to hospital.
Care of the dying and the bereaved.

The course should include experience of nursing people of all age groups and, although participation in a primary care team may be difficult to arrange, promotion of health and preventive care should be emphasised wherever relevant in all areas of practice.

Appendix D: Content analysis of student timetables

Table D1 Analysis of foundation unit and medical module timetables according to categories of sessions

Category of session	Module									Total	%
	FU	M1	M1	M3	M3	12	13	14	15		
Medical speciality any session with reference to medical speciality, specific disease	1	6	6	4	8	10	7	7	7	56	23
Biological science anatomy, physiology, pathology, nutrition, pharmacology	31	3	1	6	5	3	2	4	4	59	24
Technical procedures e.g. radiotherapy, X-ray and ultrasound	6	3	1	2	1	0	0	0	1	14	6
Nursing procedures e.g. bedbaths, mouth care, patient handling	23	14	1	0	0	1	0	1	2	42	18
Affective/psychosocial nursing e.g. listening and interviewing skills, discussion of critical incidents, patients in pain, death, dying, perceptions of patients' behaviour	5	1	3	4	3	4*	2	2	0	24	10
Activities of daily living & functional disorders e.g. assisting patients with ADLs; rehabilitation, care of unconscious/dyspnoeic patients	2	3	1	0	0	1	0	0	1	8	3
Nursing process	1	1	0	0	0	0	0	0	0	2	1
Ward–school interface e.g. discussion of ward experiences	11	2	1	0	2	1	0	0	0	17	7
Guided study work sheets, library	5	3	0	0	0	0	1	0	3	12	5
Individual study	3	0	0	0	0	1	1	1	0	6	3
Total										240	100

* Plus additional sessions in an oncology study day

Appendix E: Findings from the ward learning environment student rating questionnaire

Table E1 Work and other experiences identified as valuable to education: patient characteristics (12 medical wards, 79 questionnaire respondents, 158 comments)

Valuable educational experiences	No. of comments
Caring for:	
Elderly mentally infirm patients	4
Women patients	1
Elderly patients	1
Total	**6**

Table E2 Work and other experiences identified as valuable to education: basic nursing (12 medical wards, 79 questionnaire respondents, 158 comments)

Valuable educational experiences	No. of comments
Basic/general/routine	9
Heavy work	2
Night duty	1
Last offices	1
Severely ill patient	1
Unconscious patient	1
Total	**15**

Table E3 Work and other experiences identified as valuable to education: technical nursing (12 medical wards, 79 questionnaire respondents, 158 comments)

Valuable educational experiences	No. of comments
Chemotherapy and radiotherapy	7
Barrier nursing	4
Observations (e.g. temperature, pulse, respiration, blood pressure)	3
Surgical dressings	2
Cardiac arrest/emergency	2
Drug rounds	1
Injections	1
Intravenous antibiotics	1
ECGs and cardiac monitoring	1
Underwater seal drainage	1
Tracheostomy and airway	1
Unspecified procedures	2
Total	26

Table E4 Work and other experiences identified as valuable to education: affective nursing (3 oncology wards and 9 other medical wards, 79 questionnaire respondents, 158 comments)

Valuable educational experiences	No. of comments	
	Oncology wards	Other medical wards
Terminal care of patients including relatives	7	5
Talking to patients	3	0
Pain control	2	0
Coping with patients' and relatives' grief	1	0
Psychological care of oncology patients	1	0
Care of aggressive/ violent/confused patients	0	5
Total	14	10
Grand total (all wards)	24	

Table E5 Work and other experiences identified as valuable to education: specialist medical knowledge, investigations and treatment (12 medical wards, 79 questionnaire respondents, 158 comments)

Valuable educational experiences	No. of comments
Observation of medical investigations e.g. cardiac catheterisation, endoscopy, bronchoscopy	17
Cardiology	3
Diabetes	1
Oncological disease processes	1
Rare diseases	1
Neurological diseases	1
Anatomy and physiology of the brain	1
Acute surgical patient	1
Patient with jaundice	1
Patient with tuberculosis in isolation	1
Patient with acute respiratory disease	1
Total	29

Table E6(a) Students' ratings of 12 medical wards on item 36: frequency of experiencing anxiety or stress

Ward	Number	Mean	S.D.
1. Kinder	51	2.24	0.68
2. Ronda	52	2.10	0.89
3. Windermere	43	1.56	0.77
4. Edale	48	1.44	0.80
5. Langdale	29	1.55	0.69
6. Ullswater	50	1.74	0.72
7. Coniston	38	1.53	0.86
8. Ambleside	47	1.62	0.90
9. Loughrigg	62	1.82	0.78
10. Eskdale	35	1.71	0.75
11. Buttermere	35	2.23	0.69
12. Wastwater	34	2.21	0.69

Maximum score 3, minimum 0.

Table E6(b) Gabriel's test of significance at the 0.05 level for comparison between scores obtained on item 36

	1	2	3	4	5	6	7	8	9	10	11
2	N										
3	S	S									
4	S	S	N								
5	S	S	N	N							
6	S	S	N	N	N						
7	S	S	N	N	N	N					
8	S	S	N	N	N	N	N				
9	S	S	N	N	N	N	N	N			
10	S	S	N	N	N	N	N	N	N		
11	N	N	S	S	S	S	S	S	S	S	
12	N	N	S	S	S	S	S	S	S	S	N

S = significant at the 0.05 level
N = not significant

182

Table E7(a) Students' ratings of 12 medical wards on Section E: patient care

Ward	Number	Mean	S.D.
1. Edale	48	4.28	0.47
2. Eskdale	35	4.30	0.52
3. Wastwater	34	4.35	0.59
4. Windermere	43	4.19	0.56
5. Kinder	51	4.11	0.57
6. Buttermere	35	4.38	0.60
7. Ambleside	47	4.16	0.60
8. Langdale	29	4.20	0.66
9. Coniston	38	4.01	0.65
10. Ronda	52	4.34	0.55
11. Loughrigg	62	3.79	0.68
12. Ullswater	50	3.63	0.77

Table E7(b) Gabriel's test of significance at the 0.05 level for comparison between scores obtained on Section E

	1	2	3	4	5	6	7	8	9	10	11
2	N										
3	N	N									
4	N	N	N								
5	N	N	N	N							
6	N	N	N	N	N						
7	N	N	N	N	N	N					
8	N	N	N	N	N	N	N				
9	N	N	N	N	N	N	N	N			
10	N	N	N	N	N	N	N	N	N		
11	S	S	S	S	S	S	S	S	S	S	
12	S	S	S	S	S	S	S	S	S	S	S

S = significant at the 0.05 level
N = not significant

183

Table E8(a) Students' overall ratings of 12 medical wards as learning environments

Ward	Ward specialty & patient characteristics	Number	Mean	S.D.
1. Edale	Cardiology – female	48	3.78	0.37
2. Eskdale	Oncology – female	35	3.64	0.40
3. Wastwater	Oncology – male	34	3.64	0.51
4. Windermere	Gastroenterology – m/f	43	3.57	0.43
5. Kinder	Endocrinology – male	51	3.52	0.50
6. Buttermere	Oncology – female	35	3.51	0.54
7. Ambleside	Cardiology – male	47	3.47	0.58
8. Langdale	Endocrinology – 'heavy' elderly female population	29	3.46	0.46
9. Coniston	Gastroenterology – 'heavy' elderly female population	38	3.44	0.47
10. Ronda	Respiratory medicine – 'heavy' elderly f. pop.	52	3.41	0.40
11. Loughrigg	Neurology – male/female	62	3.11	0.52
12. Ullswater	Respiratory medicine – male	50	3.01	0.48

Table E8(b) Gabriel's test of significance at the 0.05 level for comparison between overall ratings for pairs of wards

	1	2	3	4	5	6	7	8	9	10	11
2	N										
3	N	N									
4	N	N	N								
5	S	N	N	N							
6	S	N	N	N	N						
7	S	N	N	N	N	N					
8	S	N	N	N	N	N	N				
9	S	N	N	N	N	N	N	N			
10	S	N	N	N	N	N	N	N	N		
11	S	S	S	S	S	S	S	S	S	S	
12	S	S	S	S	S	S	S	S	S	S	N

S = significant at the 0.05 level
N = not significant

Table E9(a) Students' ratings of 12 medical wards on Section C: ward teaching

Ward	Number	Mean	S.D.
1. Edale	48	3.49	0.52
2. Eskdale	35	3.12	0.62
3. Wastwater	34	3.34	0.61
4. Windermere	43	2.84	0.51
5. Kinder	51	3.36	0.57
6. Buttermere	35	3.04	0.62
7. Ambleside	47	2.93	0.75
8. Langdale	29	2.82	0.60
9. Coniston	38	2.61	0.54
10. Ronda	52	2.70	0.62
11. Loughrigg	62	2.54	0.61
12. Ullswater	50	2.36	0.60

Table E9(b) Gabriel's test of significance at the 0.05 level for comparison between scores obtained on Section C

	1	2	3	4	5	6	7	8	9	10	11
2	S										
3	N	S									
4	S	N	S								
5	N	S	N	S							
6	S	N	S	N	S						
7	S	N	S	N	S	N					
8	S	N	S	N	S	N	N				
9	S	S	S	N	S	S	S	N			
10	S	S	S	N	S	S	N	N	N		
11	S	S	S	S	S	S	S	N	N	N	
12	S	S	S	S	S	S	S	S	S	S	S

S = significant at the 0.05 level
N = not significant

Table E10(a) Students' ratings of 12 medical wards on Section D: provision of learning opportunities

Ward	Number	Mean	S.D.
1. Edale	48	3.09	0.44
2. Eskdale	35	2.78	0.51
3. Wastwater	34	2.80	0.56
4. Windermere	43	2.89	0.42
5. Kinder	51	2.95	0.50
6. Buttermere	35	2.71	0.64
7. Ambleside	47	2.80	0.60
8. Langdale	29	2.79	0.51
9. Coniston	38	2.77	0.42
10. Ronda	52	2.80	0.56
11. Loughrigg	62	2.43	0.49
12. Ullswater	50	2.32	0.50

Table E10(b) Gabriel's test of significance at the 0.05 level for comparison between scores obtained on Section D

	1	2	3	4	5	6	7	8	9	10	11
2	S										
3	S	N									
4	S	N	N								
5	S	N	N	N							
6	S	N	N	N	N						
7	S	N	N	N	N	N					
8	S	N	N	N	N	N	N				
9	S	N	N	N	N	N	N	N			
10	S	N	N	N	N	N	N	N	N		
11	S	S	S	S	S	S	S	S	S	S	
12	S	S	S	S	S	S	S	S	S	S	N

S = significant at the 0.05 level
N = not significant

186

Table E11(a)   Students' ratings of 12 medical wards on
Section B: ward atmosphere/staff relations

Ward	Number	Mean	S.D.
1. Edale	48	3.93	0.64
2. Eskdale	35	3.91	0.71
3. Wastwater	34	3.81	0.85
4. Windermere	43	3.99	0.87
5. Kinder	51	3.59	0.80
6. Buttermere	35	3.70	0.97
7. Ambleside	47	3.42	0.96
8. Langdale	29	4.00	0.68
9. Coniston	38	4.19	0.62
10. Ronda	52	4.33	0.58
11. Loughrigg	62	3.11	0.87
12. Ullswater	50	3.21	0.76

Table E11(b)   Gabriel's test of significance at the 0.05 level for
comparison between scores obtained on Section
B

	1	2	3	4	5	6	7	8	9	10	11
2	N										
3	N	N									
4	N	N	N								
5	N	N	N	N							
6	N	N	N	N	N						
7	S	S	S	S	N	N					
8	N	N	N	N	N	N	S				
9	N	N	N	N	S	N	S	N			
10	S	S	S	S	S	S	S	N	N		
11	S	S	S	S	S	S	S	S	S	S	
12	S	S	S	S	S	S	N	S	S	S	N

S = significant at the 0.05 level
N = not significant

Table E12(a) Module 1 students' overall ratings of 12 medical wards as learning environments

Ward	Number	Mean	S.D.
1. Edale	17	3.90	0.34
2. Eskdale	7	3.86	0.23
3. Wastwater	6	3.96	0.33
4. Windermere	14	3.71	0.28
5. Kinder	15	3.86	0.36
6. Buttermere	7	3.91	0.25
7. Ambleside	15	3.58	0.53
8. Langdale	11	3.46	0.45
9. Coniston	13	3.58	0.35
10. Ronda	16	3.45	0.34
11. Loughrigg	8	3.68	0.42
12. Ullswater	13	3.28	0.34

Range of scores: 3.96–3.28

Table E12(b) Gabriel's test of significance at the 0.05 level for comparison between scores obtained from Module 1 students

	1	2	3	4	5	6	7	8	9	10	11
2	N										
3	N	N									
4	N	N	N								
5	N	N	N	N							
6	N	N	N	N	N						
7	N	N	N	N	N	N					
8	S	N	N	N	N	N	N				
9	N	N	N	N	N	N	N	N			
10	S	N	S	N	S	N	N	N	N		
11	N	N	N	N	N	N	N	N	N	N	
12	S	S	S	S	S	S	N	N	N	N	N

S = significant at the 0.05 level
N = not significant

188

Table E13(a) Module 3 students' overall ratings of 12 medical wards as learning environments

Ward	Number	Mean	S.D.
1. Edale	11	3.85	0.29
2. Eskdale	10	3.83	0.38
3. Wastwater	11	3.88	0.27
4. Windermere	11	3.66	0.41
5. Kinder	11	3.66	0.47
6. Buttermere	8	3.49	0.53
7. Ambleside	12	3.41	0.73
8. Langdale	6	3.60	0.42
9. Coniston	10	3.39	0.35
10. Ronda	11	3.46	0.62
11. Loughrigg	13	3.04	0.51
12. Ullswater	11	2.84	0.50

Range of scores: 3.88–2.84

Table E13(b) Gabriel's test of significance at the 0.05 level for comparison between scores obtained from Module 3 students

	1	2	3	4	5	6	7	8	9	10	11
2	N										
3	N	N									
4	N	N	N								
5	N	N	N	N							
6	N	N	N	N	N						
7	N	N	N	N	N	N					
8	N	N	N	N	N	N	N				
9	N	N	N	N	N	N	N	N			
10	N	N	N	N	N	N	N	N	N		
11	S	S	S	S	S	N	N	N	N	N	
12	S	S	S	S	S	S	S	S	S	S	N

S = significant at the 0.05 level
N = not significant

189

Table E14(a) Module 12 students' overall ratings of 12 medical wards as learning environments

Ward	Number	Mean	S.D.
1. Edale	8	3.62	0.35
2. Eskdale	8	3.56	0.36
3. Wastwater	6	3.37	0.54
4. Windermere	9	3.46	0.55
5. Kinder	10	3.23	0.55
6. Buttermere	9	3.23	0.65
7. Ambleside	12	3.20	0.47
8. Langdale	6	3.23	0.39
9. Coniston	9	3.53	0.64
10. Ronda	11	3.27	0.36
11. Loughrigg	18	2.85	0.49
12. Ullswater	12	3.00	0.60

Range of scores: 3.62–2.85

Table E14(b) Gabriel's test of significance at the 0.05 level for comparison between scores obtained from Module 12 students

	1	2	3	4	5	6	7	8	9	10	11
2	N										
3	N	N									
4	N	N	N								
5	N	N	N	N							
6	N	N	N	N	N						
7	N	N	N	N	N	N					
8	N	N	N	N	N	N	N				
9	N	N	N	N	N	N	N	N			
10	N	N	N	N	N	N	N	N	N		
11	S	N	N	N	N	N	N	N	N	N	
12	N	N	N	N	N	N	N	N	N	N	N

S = significant at the 0.05 level
N = not significant

190

Table E15(a) Module 14 students' overall ratings of 12 medical wards as learning environments

Ward	Number	Mean	S.D.
1. Edale	12	3.63	0.45
2. Eskdale	10	3.37	0.39
3. Wastwater	11	3.37	0.59
4. Windermere	9	3.35	0.45
5. Kinder	15	3.27	0.37
6. Buttermere	11	3.51	0.51
7. Ambleside	8	3.74	0.45
8. Langdale	6	3.52	0.62
9. Coniston	6	3.12	0.56
10. Ronda	14	3.42	0.29
11. Loughrigg	23	3.15	0.44
12. Ullswater	14	2.89	0.40

Range of scores: 3.74–2.89

Table E15(b) Gabriel's test of significance at the 0.05 level for comparison between scores obtained from Module 14 students

	1	2	3	4	5	6	7	8	9	10	11
2	N										
3	N	N									
4	N	N	N								
5	N	N	N	N							
6	N	N	N	N	N						
7	N	N	N	N	N	N					
8	N	N	N	N	N	N	N				
9	N	N	N	N	N	N	N	N			
10	N	N	N	N	N	N	N	N	N		
11	N	N	N	N	N	N	N	N	N	N	
12	S	S	S	S	N	S	S	S	N	S	N

S = significant at the 0.05 level
N = not significant

191

Table E16(a) Students' ratings of 12 medical wards on Item 2: 'I am happy with the experience I have had on this ward'

Ward	Number	Mean	S.D.
1. Edale	48	4.32	0.66
2. Eskdale	35	4.23	0.76
3. Wastwater	34	4.12	0.80
4. Windermere	43	4.16	0.80
5. Kinder	51	3.82	1.01
6. Buttermere	35	3.80	1.19
7. Ambleside	47	3.98	0.96
8. Langdale	29	3.97	1.03
9. Coniston	38	4.13	0.95
10. Ronda	52	3.98	0.89
11. Loughrigg	62	3.63	1.14
12. Ullswater	50	3.60	0.96

Table E16(b) Gabriel's test of significance at the 0.05 level for comparison between scores obtained on Item 2

	1	2	3	4	5	6	7	8	9	10	11
2	N										
3	N	N									
4	N	N	N								
5	N	N	N	N							
6	N	N	N	N	N						
7	N	N	N	N	N	N					
8	N	N	N	N	N	N	N				
9	N	N	N	N	N	N	N	N			
10	N	N	N	N	N	N	N	N	N		
11	S	S	N	N	N	N	N	N	N	N	
12	S	N	N	N	N	N	N	N	N	N	N

S = significant at the 0.05 level
N = not significant

Notes

Chapter 1

1.   Evidence of 'lack of care' in long-stay institutions includes a study of work organisation and social relations in a geriatric hospital (Evers, 1981a, 1984). The findings of a number of studies quoted by Evers summarise life in a geriatric hospital as routinised physical care; harassed nurses battling against the clock; depersonalisation of patients to the status of work objects. Evers uses the notion of 'warehousing' to analyse patterns of work organisation on different wards. 'Warehousing', i.e. care at its most routine and depersonalised, as distinct from a 'horticultural' model which encourages individuality, was first conceptualised by Miller and Gwynne (1972) in a study of institutional care for the disabled. Evers describes 'minimal' warehousing wards where patients were subject to indiscriminate routines and institutional clothing. On 'personalised' warehousing wards (no wards practised a horticultural model of care), patients were 'lovingly' cared for and had their own clothing, hairstyles, hearing aids, spectacles and dentures. Incidents of 'inhumane' treatment were less likely on these wards. Inhumane treatment was defined by Evers as primary (ignoring patients), secondary (lack of response to patients' distress); tertiary (making decisions for patients in their absence).

2.   The 'little things' are the victims of what Davies (1990) and other writers call competing rationalities which underpin institutionalised care work. Scientific and technical–economic rationalities correspond to male-orientated doctor and administrator 'assembly line care of the sick'. Costs are kept to a minimum and as many patients as possible are processed through medical diagnosis and treatment in the minimum time possible. Female

caring activities are motivated by a responsibility or nurturing rationality where 'response to human need', often through the so-called 'little things,' is paramount. In institutionalised care, however, where scientific and technical–economic rationalities dominate, these 'little things' are neither recognised nor costed into the work process except by the carers who struggle to 'fit them in'. The moral and ethical dimensions of caring and the controversial question as to whether women develop a gender-specific morality are considered by Gilligan (1982) and Tronto (1987).

3. Abel-Smith (1960) suggests that nursing in the voluntary hospitals provided a suitable occupation for the daughters of the higher social classes. It was only able to do this however by promoting nursing as a 'vocation' requiring duty, devotion and obedience, the epitome of the 'good' woman. In keeping with the social relationships of Victorian middle-class society, nurses (women) were expected to be subordinate to doctors (men). I found a quotation written by a *Daily Telegraph* correspondent sometime in 1888 which stated quite categorically that women should behave in a way that recognised they were inferior to men. The correspondent wrote: 'No sensible woman objects to acknowledging what is the fact, that she is physically and intellectually inferior to men'.

See also Carpenter (1978) and Gamarnikow (1978) for descriptions of the reproduction of the patriarchal family structure in the voluntary hospitals between doctors–matrons–nurses and doctors–nurses–patients.

Carpenter (1978) suggests that 'what emerged in the voluntary hospital was the reproduction of the wider Victorian class structure based on preconceived notions of the division of labour between the sexes and between women of different classes'. The ward sister or matron complemented the authority of the doctor (a man) in organising the nurses and domestic staff in a mirror image of how, as the 'lady of the house', she would have supported her husband and supervised the servants.

Of particular interest is Gamarnikow's point that because nursing occupies a role in subordination to medicine, doctors are in sole charge of who is defined as a patient. The nurse–doctor–patient relationship mirrors the power relations between men, women and children within the patriarchal family.

4. Ungerson (1983*a*) draws attention to women's unpaid and unrecognised contribution to the maintenance of the British Welfare State. Ungerson describes how women may be involved throughout their lives in caring for others: a child, a husband, a sick, handicapped or elderly relative in a 'cycle of care'.

5. Ungerson (1983*b*), in line with others, claims that women have a set of skills unique to their gender. Mothering as an example of 'private' care work has much in common with institutionalised, i.e. 'public', care work. Ungerson itemises these skills in the following way:

(a) Time available at short notice and in flexible lumps;
(b) High levels of skill in domestic tasks – e.g. cooking, cleaning, washing;
(c) High levels of social skill, for example talking and listening in order to assess present and future needs;
(d) Skills in information gathering about other services and ability to act autonomously over a wide range of tasks of widely differing skill level;
(e) Punctuality and reliability;
(f) Ability to operate over long periods in fairly isolated circumstances, engaging in routine and often unpleasant tasks, particularly in the case of the very old, the mentally handicapped and mentally ill – very little measurable 'success' and positive response from recipients.

Ungerson refers to these items as the 'socially expected attributes of women' in Western Europe. They also comprehensively describe the attributes expected of nurses and give insights into the nature of nursing.

Davies and Rosser (1986), in a study of women working as Higher Clerical officers in the health service, introduce the term 'gendered job' to describe how gender is built into the labour process. The job 'capitalises on the qualities and capabilities a woman has gained by virtue of having lived her life as a woman'. But, like nurses, these qualities and capabilities were regarded as part of the package rather than as an essential part of the job requiring higher status and financial rewards.

6. The nursing process has two components: the underlying philosophy that promotes a people-orientated approach to patients based on models of care such as Henderson's (1960), and Roper's (1976) living activities and a problem-solving work method. The nursing process as work method recommends the organisation of nursing into four stages defined as assessment, planning, implementation and evaluation of patient care.

McFarlane (1977) in her keynote address clearly spelt out the skills that nurses would require to practise the 'process' effectively. The observational and interviewing skills spelt out by McFarlane were clearly 'people' skills, the acquisition of which was necessary if the nursing process was to become part of the nurse's 'approach and repertoire'. In the same year (1977), the nursing process appeared for the first time in the syllabus of the national nurse training curriculum (General Nursing Council, 1977). Armstrong (1983) noted that once the nursing process had become officialised in this way, the textbook presentation of the nurse's role changed. Patients were no longer described in strictly biological terms. Psychology and communication skills were emphasised and 'subjectivity' and emotions were encouraged as part of the nurse–patient relationship.

The introduction of the nursing process, with its emphasis on emotional care, has seen a rapid increase of nursing textbooks and videotapes dealing with the teaching of interpersonal and communication skills. The development of good nurse–patient relationships was hailed as therapeutic and central to the healing process.

For comprehensive reviews of the nursing process, see De la Cuesta (1979, 1983); Brooking (1986).

Theoretical limitations of the nursing process have been exposed by a number of writers (Roper et al., 1985). A variety of nursing theories and models are being offered to create an informed base for the use of the nursing process (Aggleton and Chalmers, 1986; see also Salvage and Kershaw, 1990).

7.   According to Salvage (1990) the 'New Nursing' dates back to the 1970s. She identifies a number of influences which have contributed to its development: the growth of academic departments of nursing with a fresh interest in nursing theories, the challenge of the women's movement to male (i.e. doctor) subordination and the influence of the Americans in redefining the nurse's unique contribution to healing. Salvage summarises an important element of the new nursing ideology and practice as 'transforming relationships with patients – away

196

from the biomedical model which views medical intervention as the solution to health problems, towards a holistic approach promoting the patient's active participation in care'. Quoting Pearson (1988), primary nursing, in which a nurse is assigned to care for a patient from admission to discharge, is seen as ideally suited to developing close therapeutic relationships.

Salvage also mentions a number of other nursing innovations including Nursing Development Units and the setting up of nursing beds into which nurses rather than doctors admit and care for patients.

8. Freidson (1970) suggests that nurses can never be completely professionally autonomous, because traditionally their knowledge and skills revolve around the diagnostic and treatment model of cure. As discussed in note 3 above, doctors also control the admission of patients and their treatment. In the public's eyes nurses are seen as doctors' assistants. They also rely on being part of the medical division of labour for their claims to being professional. As described in notes 6 and 7, nurses are seeking their own knowledge base and work methods based on alternative paradigms of healing, holism and emotional care in order to free themselves from medical dominance. A recent article in the *Nursing Standard* suggests that they have enjoyed only limited success (Hand, 1991).

9. Salvage describes *The Politics of Nursing* as the product of years of informal and formal discussion with nurses and participation in groups such as the Radical Nurses in the early 1980s. I was a member of the group at the time and we wanted desperately to offer an alternative analysis to mainstream views of nursing and nurses as meek, submissive and mindless.

10. Mary O'Brien (1989) defines 'male-stream' thought as 'the massive dense intellectual current of male intellectual history' as opposed to the relatively short public history of feminist understanding (p.3) which allows women to reproduce the world in their own terms. Male-stream thought and the belief that knowledge is 'objective' and 'abstract', promotes dualism and the setting up of opposites in a systematic way. Hence mind is described as abstract, body as material; science as abstract,

common sense as material; intellectual work as abstract, manual and domestic labour as material; male as abstract, female as material and so on (p.7).

11. Some feminists/sociologists (Knights and Morgan, 1990; Shaw, 1990) take issue with the use of the word 'strategy' because of its male, military connotations. Its use may presuppose that individuals have clear goals and objectives in mind when they decide how they will behave. Although I accept that this is not always the case I would argue that individuals are not passive victims shaped inevitably by circumstances and people, but have the capacity to take control over their lives. In a hierarchically structured environment such as nursing, the use of the word strategy seems particularly appropriate to describe ways in which nurses control and make choices about their social relations. Indeed, the women's movement has contributed greatly to this view through consciousness raising groups as a means of empowering women. If the issue over the use of the word (strategy) is one of semantics then I accept the need to seek new terminologies generated from the data and grounded in people's own words.

Chapter 2

1. See Beardshaw and Robinson (1990), Section 1, pp. 8–12, for an analysis of the nursing workforce accompanied by a series of Department of Health graphs. Since 1979, there has been a steady but modest increase of staff, especially amongst registered nurses and health visitors. This increase, however, has not kept pace with workload. The number of nursing students has declined dramatically. The reasons for the decline were not only to do with fewer 18 year old females in the population from whom nurses had traditionally been recruited, but fewer women choosing nursing as a career. The DoH's decision to phase out the two-year pupil nurse training programme (see below) also contributed to the falling number of trainees.

2. Until the phasing out of pupil nurse training during the 1980s, in line with the Project 2000 recommendation that there should be a single level of registered nurse, trainees could choose between two training schemes. Pupil nurse training took two years and prepared nurses for the roll. Student nurse training took three years and prepared nurses for the register. Career prospects for enrolled nurses were limited, although in effect many of them have undertaken the same work as registered nurses, but for less pay and status. Entry requirements differed for the two schemes in that pupils were not required to be so 'academically' qualified as students. In effect, what this meant was that pupil nurse training was more likely to be offered to working class and/or recruits from black and ethnic minority groups, including overseas applicants.

The last group of pupil nurses had completed their training at the 'City' Hospital just before I commenced my study.

3.   'City' Hospital and school of nursing is a pseudonym, as are all other such proper names used in the study.

4.   See Cole (1987) and Platzer (1988) for a discussion of racial and sexual discrimination in nursing recruitment and retention. See also *BMJ* editorial on black nurses, September (1988) and Hicks' (1982) study of racism in nursing.

5.   During the 1960s, a minimum of two Ordinary Level certificates of general education (GCE) were required for those undertaking training for the register. The teaching hospitals, however, had a tradition of demanding higher qualifications ranging from five 'O levels' to two Advanced Level certificates in some institutions. Recruitment has now been centralised through a central clearing house. A minimum of five Ordinary Level certificates of secondary education are required (GCSE), but when I rang up to enquire about becoming a nurse I was told that I could sit a special entry test if I didn't have the formal entry qualifications necessary. This has always been the case, even in the days of two certificate entry.

6.   See note 8, Chapter 1

7.   See note 4 above.

8.   Training Body and inspectorate: The General Nursing Council of England and Wales was founded in 1919 to administer nurse training and professional practice. The standard

ward based assessment procedures similar to those undertaken by the City nurses are outlined in GNC Communication 69/4/3 Paper C (1969): Changes proposed in the Final State Examination. In 1983, the Council's functions were taken over by the United Kingdom Central Council for Nursing, Midwifery and Health Visiting and four national boards, including the English National Board.

9. See note 5, Chapter 1, on women's socially expected attributes.

Chapter 3

1. See note 7, Chapter 1, on the 'New Nursing'.

2. See note 6, Chapter 1, on the nursing process as philosophy and work method.

3. As in note 2 above.

4. During critical incident sessions, students drew on incidents from their ward experiences in order to learn about about their feelings, behaviour and attitudes. The underlying assumption of the technique was that, by exploring in detail incidents from their daily work, the students could assess the influence their attitudes had on standards of care.

5. Since January 1981, all general nursing students must spend an 8–12 week allocation in psychiatric nursing. Research shows that in the short-term, students gain confidence in their abilities to recognise and care for patients with mental illness. However, Collister (1983) found that only four months later, when the students had returned to general nursing, these abilities were lost. The problems of applying and reinforcing skills learnt in the psychiatric setting to the general wards arise because of the diversity of the two cultures.

An unpublished study undertaken at a neighbouring teaching hospital shortly after I had completed data collection confirmed the findings of previous research. During their psychiatric placement, students were able to identify various skills they had learned. A group of third-year students who had completed

200

their psychiatric placement one year previously could only identify talking to patients and dealing with aggression as skills they had learnt. The students on placement were much more specific and identified listening skills, non-verbal communication, empathy and observational skills, such as looking for signs of anxiety in patients. They were keen to take these skills back to general nursing, but thought that there might be pressure from qualified staff not to spend time talking to patients. The third-year students, whilst acknowledging that patients on general wards had psychological needs, felt that physical needs were more important and that there wasn't enough time to talk with patients (quoted from unpublished report).

6.   The students tended to see knowledge as facts that had to be formally taught, which were different to what they did. Collins (1974) and Eraut (1985) offer alternative approaches to conceptualising knowledge and the teaching–learning process which are more appropriate to the students' accounts of so-called natural skills and informal learning. Collins does not regard knowledge as entirely 'pure' (cf. O'Brien, on 'abstract' knowledge, note 10, Chapter 1). Knowledge also consists of unformulated tacit rules. The language student, for example, not only acquires knowledge but also builds up tacit understanding during the learning process. Eraut distinguishes between technical knowledge, which is written and codified, and practical knowledge, which is expressed only in practice and learned through 'doing'. Practical knowledge is uncodified and transmitted through tone, feel and expression (Eraut, 1985, p.119), like the students accounts of *just* learning, 'picking up', 'watching', a set of hitherto uncodified caring skills.

7.   The idea of teaching nurses to care always evokes a heated reaction, for a number of reasons. Nurses and others are concerned that by learning to manage feelings they will appear false and insincere. Hochschild (1983) is also uncomfortable about the content of the training programmes on emotional labour, to which the flight attendants were exposed. She observed that, potentially, these training programmes de-skilled the flight attendants in that their personal repertoire of feelings and reactions in encounters with passengers became circumscribed by their training programmes. Instead of reacting spontaneously to a given situation 'the overall definition of the

task is more rigid and the worker's field of choice about what to do is greatly narrowed' (p.120).

Chapter 4

1. Traditionally, student nurse allocation has been based on medical specialties. Roper (1975) undertook a study to examine the clinical content of the areas to which students were allocated. She observed both students and patients, and examined the nursing records in order to establish the learning content available on each ward. Roper discovered that sometimes patients' diagnostic labels were different from the designated specialty of the ward. It also appeared that any patient, irrespective of diagnosis, provided nurses with teaching and learning. Roper concluded that it was difficult to predict learning experience on the basis of medical specialty. She decided therefore to develop a patient profile instrument based on Henderson's (1960) living activities. She showed how her instrument could be used as an alternative to medical diagnosis to define student learning and to plan allocation related to patient dependency and nursing needs.

2. Fretwell (1982) found a similar pecking order in the students' ratings of their learning environments according to medical specialties.

3. Experimental forms of nurse training have been in operation since the 1950s, including a number of university and polytechnic programmes (MacGuire, 1980). I was a student on one of these undergraduate programmes in the late 1960s. The content and structure of the course promoted a holistic and integrated approach to health care. Even so, the practice I encountered on the wards was medically driven. Despite the 'New Nursing' (see note 7, Chapter 1) the situation showed little change when in the mid-1980s I supervised undergraduate nursing students in the clinical areas.

4. These are similar findings to those of Melia (1982), Fretwell (1982) and Alexander (1983) who found that students categorised 'basic nursing' as low status work with little learning

value. 'Technical nursing' had high prestige and learning value. Melia found that students classified 'patients' who required predominantly 'social' care as 'not really nursing'.

5.   Strauss and colleagues (1982b) describe how medical legitimisation shapes the nature of the work that nurses and others do in the 'technologised hospital'. Different tasks are distributed amongst workers, and involve two types of relationships: one is instrumental, for carrying out physical and technical tasks with the patient; the other is expressive, concerning patients' psychosocial care. Strauss and colleagues have coined the term 'sentimental work' to describe and specify the content of 'psychosocial care'.

Sentimental work is defined as an ingredient of any kind of work where the object being worked on is alive, sentient and reacting. The nature of sentimental work changed according to what was wrong with the patient, their individual illness trajectory and the predominant ward ethos. Sentimental work was circumscribed by the medical specialty of the ward, although 'there are moments and phases in trajectories' such as terminal illness 'when the staff recognise this work is very pertinent'.

Seven categories of sentimental work were generated from data collected during field observations and interviews. Strauss and colleagues suggest their typology is useful for specifying the 'conditions, consequences and tactics' of the much used but vague term of 'working psychologically' with patients. Nurses are more likely to undertake certain types of sentimental work. As staff were not held accountable for doing sentimental work, nor was it necessarily an ingredient of trajectory work, the work was often carried out on an *ad hoc* basis. Unless it was documented or verbally reported, sentimental work remained invisible.

6.   In an extensive critique of the literature on 'good' and 'bad' patients, Kelly and May (1982) also found that patients with certain illnesses, diseases and symptoms were more or less popular with doctors and nurses. Their popularity also depended on their age, gender, race and class characteristics. The most popular patients were young and suffering from curable illnesses which responded to specific medical and nursing skills. See also Stockwell, 1972.

Kelly and May found that the notion of a 'caring' nurse was dependent on the notion of an 'appreciative' patient, one who confirmed the role of the nurse. Patients who denied that legitimisation were seen as 'bad patients'.

In relation to the present study, this observation is important, since it suggests that students found it easier to undertake emotional labour, i.e. appear more caring, towards patients that they liked. The story of Mr Bear illustrates this point very clearly. Emotional labour costs less when the patient is appreciative.

7. Teaching on race, ethnicity and culture was relatively weak at the City Hospital during the period of the study. This improved slightly following the introduction of an equal opportunities policy. Despite the more people-centred approach of Project 2000, there is still some criticism of nurse education in general for its lack of attention to race and ethnicity within the curriculum. See Mohammed (1986).

Chapter 5

1. See note 2, Chapter 1.

2. See discussion on Menzies (1960), Chapter 1.

3. As for note 1 above.

4. Davies (1990) says that male notions of time (see note 2, Chapter 1) are inappropriate to care work. Flexible timetables are required to allow carers to respond to individuals' ever changing needs.

5. See note 1, Chapter 1.

6. Fretwell categorised the ward sisters in her study according to their preferences and priorities. She developed a typology according to whether the sister organised her work around doctors (cf. scientific rationality), administration (cf. technical–economic rationality) or patients (cf. nurturing rationality). Those sisters who were more patient-centred also tended to be more interested in student teaching.

7.   As for note 2 above.

Chapter 6

1.   I was aware of and had read a number of studies about dying before I wrote this chapter. These studies included Glaser and Strauss's (1965, 1970) work: *Awareness of dying* and *Anguish: a case history of a dying trajectory,* and David Field's *Nursing the dying* (1989). I also talked to Nicky James and read her work on hospice care. All are fine works and undoubtedly heightened my sensitivity and drew my attention to particular aspects of death and dying in hospital. For example, Glaser and Strauss (1965, 1970) address three key issues which are apparent in the structure of my chapter: (1) how death and dying are defined in hospital and the uncertainty surrounding if, when and how it will occur; (2) how the patient's dying trajectory is systematised and managed by hospital personnel given the unpredictability of death (patients can alternate between 'certain to die on time' and 'lingering reprieve'); and (3) accountable and non-accountable aspects of terminal care. Nurses were held accountable for physical care, observation of vital signs and pain relief, which often increased as death approached. No member of staff was held accountable for psychosocial aspects of care, with the result that the 'demanding' patient of their case study became more isolated as death approached.

2.   Glaser and Strauss's notion of sentimental (see note 5, Chapter 4) order, for example, is very important in terms of how the feeling rules of a ward are shaped by the medical as well as the nursing agenda. The sentimental order is associated with the number of deaths expected to take place on a ward. Glaser and Strauss found that involvement with patients was encouraged on those wards with low expectation of death. Because death was an infrequent event and because nurses became involved with patients, they were extremely upset when any of them died. On wards which cared for cancer patients or on intensive therapy units, where the death rate was high, the sentimental order of the ward discouraged patient involvement. Nurses learnt to maintain their composure during the dying process and transfer their involvement to the patient's relatives.

Times have changed since Glaser and Strauss first reported their findings (1965). There is now a greater recognition by society in general and health carers in particular that the psychological impact of death and dying must be acknowledged, especially in oncology wards and hospices, but not necessarily on general wards.

3. This is an example of surface acting. The student said she felt sad because she thought that was how she should feel.

4. Was the student deep acting, in that, because she knew the patient, she could really feel her suffering and knew how to comfort her?

5. Benner and Wrubel (1989) believe that one way of overcoming the problem described by the patient 'i.e. to prevent getting involved', is to see people as involved in a context (p.48).

The authors draw on Heideggerian philosophy and a phenomenological perspective to view the person as neither subject nor object. The person (the nurse) through concern (an essential part of human existence) is involved in the other (the patient). This involvement means that the world is understood in the light of the concern. The person is defined by her concerns which involves her in the other. In the philosophical sense the need to prevent involvement is not an issue. But in the empirical reality, conditions may be such that the nurse is prevented from becoming involved.

Chapter 7

1. See note 5, Chapter 3.

2. See note 6, Chapter 5, on Fretwell (1982).

3. The definition of 'unstructured' comes from Ogier's (1982) study of leadership styles in ward sisters. High structure on a rating questionnaire for learners was indicative of a sister who was seen as purposeful and directive in her activities. The sister who appeared 'unstructured' received low ratings from the students because in their opinion she did not give enough purpose and direction to the work and learning on her ward.

4. Students appeared to prefer sisters with 'moderate' rather than 'high' structure because they were sufficently structured in their organisation to direct activities, but not so much as to limit learning.

5. See discussion of Menzies (1960), Chapter 1, p. 9.

6. This finding concurs with Brown (1973), who, from a study of long-stay hospital wards, concluded that only by providing strong social support could the deeply felt humanitarian views present in most hospital workers become effective and prevent the development or acceptance of beliefs that dehumanised patients.

References

Abel-Smith, B. (1960) *A History of the Nursing Profession* (London: Heinemann).

Aggleton, P. & Chalmers, H. (1986) *Nursing Models and the Nursing Process* (London: Macmillan).

Alexander, M. F. (1983) *Learning to Nurse* (Edinburgh: Churchill Livingstone).

Armstrong, D. (1983) 'The fabrication of nurse–patient relationships', *Social Science and Medicine*, 14B, 3–13.

British Medical Journal (1988) 'Black Nurses', *British Medical Journal*, 297, 639.

Beardshaw, V. & Robinson, R. (1990) *New For Old? Prospects for Nursing in the 1990s* (London: King's Fund Institute).

Bell, C. & Roberts, H. (eds) (1984) *Social Researching – Politics, Problems, Practice* (London: Routledge and Kegan Paul).

Bellaby, P. & Oribabor, P. (1980) 'The history of the present – contradiction and struggle in nursing', in Davies, C. (ed.) *Rewriting Nursing History* (London: Croom Helm).

Bendall, E. (1975) *'So you passed nurse'* (London: Royal College of Nursing).

Benner, P. (1984) *From Novice to Expert – Excellence and Power in Clinical Nursing Practice* (Menlo Park, CA: Addison-Wesley).

Benner, P. & Wrubel, R. (1989) *The Primacy of Caring: Stress and Coping in Health and Illness* (Menlo Park, CA: Addison-Wesley).

Bracken, E. & Davis, J. (1989) 'The implication of mentorship in nursing career development', *Senior Nurse*, 9, 5, 15–16.

Brindle, D. (1990) 'A happy ward with no nurses', *Guardian* 14 September.

Brooking, J. I. (1986) *Patient and Family Participation in Nursing Care: The Development of a Nursing Process Measuring Scale* (Ph.D. thesis: University of London, Kings College).

Brown, G. W. (1973) 'The mental hospital as an institution', *Social Science and Medicine*, 7, 407–24.

Bulmer, M. (1983) 'Concepts in the analysis of qualitative data', in Bulmer, M. (ed.) *Sociological Research Methods: An Introduction*, 2nd edn (London: Macmillan).

Carpenter, M. (1978) 'Managerialism and the division of labour in nursing', in Dingwall, R. & McKintosh, J. (eds) *Readings in the Sociology of Nursing* (Edinburgh: Churchill Livingstone).

Clamp, C. (1980) 'Learning through incidents', *Nursing Times*, 76, 40, 1755–8.

Cole, A. (1987) 'Racism, limited access', *Nursing Times and Nursing Mirror* 83, 24, 29–30.

Collins, H. M. (1974) 'The TEA set: Tacit knowledge and scientific networks', *Science Studies*, 4, 165–86.

Collins, H. M. (1984) 'Researching spoonbending: concepts and practice of participatory fieldwork', in Bell, C. and Roberts, H. (eds) *Social Researching – Politics, Problems, Practice* (London: Routledge and Kegan Paul).

Collister, B. (1983) 'The value of psychiatric experience in general nurse training', *Nursing Times*, Occasional Papers, 79, 29, 66–9.

Coser, R. L. (1962) *Life on the Ward* (East Lansing: Michigan State University Press).

Davies, C. (1976) 'Experience of dependency and control in work: the case of nurses', *Journal of Advanced Nursing*, 1, 273–82.

Davies, C. & Rosser, J. (1986) 'Gendered jobs in the health service: a problem for labour process analysis', in Knight, D. & Wilmott, H. (eds) *Gender and the Labour Process* (Aldershot: Gower).

Davies, K. (1990) *Women, Time and the Weavings of the Strands of Everyday Life* (Aldershot: Avebury).

De la Cuesta, C. (1979) *Nursing Process: from Theory to Implementation* (M.Sc. thesis: London University).

De la Cuesta, C. (1983) The nursing process: from development to implementation, *Journal of Advanced Nursing*, 8, 365–71.

Denzin, N. (1970) 'Strategies of multiple triangulation', in *The Research Act in Sociology* (London: Butterworth).

Department of Health (1990) *Nurse Recruitment* (London: HMSO).

Department of Health and Social Security (1972) *Report of the Committee on Nursing* (Chair: A. Briggs) (London: HMSO).

209

English National Board (1987) *Circular 1987/28/MAT*.

Eraut, M. (1985) 'Knowledge creation and knowledge use in professional contexts', *Studies in Higher Education*, 10, 2, 117–33.

Evers, H. (1981*a*) 'Tender loving care? Patients and nurses in geriatric wards', in Copp, L. A. (ed.) *Care of the Ageing* (Edinburgh: Churchill Livingstone).

Evers, H. (1981*b*) 'Care or custody? The experiences of women patients in long-stay geriatric wards', in Williams, G. & Hutter, B. (eds) *Controlling Women – the Normal and the Deviant* (London: Croom Helm).

Evers, H. K. (1984) *Patients' Experiences and Social Relations in Geriatric Wards* (Ph.D. thesis: University of Warwick).

Field, D. (1989) *Nursing the Dying* (London: Tavistock/ Routledge).

Flax, J. (1987) 'Postmodernism and gender relations in feminist theory', *Signs: Journal of Women in Culture and Society*, 12, 4, 621–43.

Freidson, E. (1970) *The Profession of Medicine: A Study of the Sociology of Applied Knowledge* (New York: Dodd, Mead and Co).

Fretwell, J. E. (1982) *Ward Teaching and Learning: Sister and the Learning Environment* (London: Royal College of Nursing).

Fretwell, J. E. (1985) *Freedom to Change* (London: Royal College of Nursing).

Gamarnikow, E. (1978) 'Sexual division of labour: the case of nursing', in Kuhn, A. & Wolpe, A. M. (eds) *Feminism and Materialism: Women and Modes of Production* (London: Routledge and Kegan Paul).

General Nursing Council Communication 69/4/3 Paper C (1969) *Changes Proposed in the Final State Examination* (London: General Nursing Council).

General Nursing Council for England and Wales (1977) *Training Syllabus. Register of Nurses: General Nursing* (London: General Nursing Council for England and Wales).

Gilligan, C. (1982) *In a Different Voice* (Cambridge MA: Harvard University Press).

Glaser, B. G. & Strauss, A. L. (1965) *Awareness of Dying* (Chicago: Aldine).

Glaser, B. & Strauss, A. (1967) *The Discovery of Grounded Theory* (London: Weidenfeld & Nicolson).

Goddard, H. A. (1953) *The Work of Nurses in Hospital Wards: Report of a Job Analysis* (Oxford: Nuffield Provincial Hospitals Trust).

Goffman, E. (1968) *Asylums* (Harmondsworth: Penguin).

Gold, R. L. (1969) 'Roles in sociological field observations', in McCall, G. J. & Simmons, J. L. (eds) *Issues in Participant Observation: a Text and Reader* (Reading MA: Addison-Wesley).

Gordon, S. (1988) 'Giving nurses time to care' *Washington Post*, 6 September.

Graham, H. (1983) 'Caring: a labour of love', in Finch, J. & Groves, D. (eds) *A Labour of Love: Women, Work and Caring* (London: Routledge and Kegan Paul).

Hand, D. (1991) 'Facts and fantasies', *Nursing Standard*, 5, 15/16, 17–19.

Hayward, J. (1975) *Information: A Prescription Against Pain* (London: Royal College of Nursing).

Henderson, V. (1960) *Basic Principles of Nursing Care* (Geneva: International Council of Nurses).

Hicks, C. (1982) 'Racism in nursing', *Nursing Times*, 78, 18, 743–8.

Hochschild, A. R. (1983) *The Managed Heart: Commercialisation of Human Feeling* (Berkeley: University of California Press).

Hochschild, A. (1989) *The Second Shift: Working Parents and the Revolution at Home* (New York: Viking/Penguin).

Huey, F. L. (1988) 'Care Plans for the USA', *American Journal of Nursing*, 1483–93.

James, N. (1984) 'A postscript to nursing', in Bell, C. & Roberts, H. (eds) *Social Researching – Politics, Problems, Practice* (London: Routledge and Kegan Paul).

James, N. (1989) 'Emotional labour, skills and work in the social regulation of feeling', *The Sociological Review*, 37, 1, 15–42.

James, V. (1986) *Care and Work in Nursing the Dying* (Ph.D. thesis: University of Aberdeen).

Johns, C. (1990) 'Autonomy of primary nurses: the need to both facilitate and limit autonomy in practice', *Journal of Advanced Nursing* 15, 886–94.

Kelly, M. P. & May, D. (1982) 'Good and bad patients: a review of the literature and a theoretical critique', *Journal of Advanced Nursing*, 7, 2, 147–57 (see particularly p. 154).

Kendall, M. G. & Stuart, A. (1968) *The Advanced Theory of Statistics*, Vol. 3, 2nd edn, pp. 43–6 (London: Charles Griffin and Co).

King, R. D., Raynes, N. V. & Tizard, J. (1971) *Patterns of Residential Care: Sociological Studies in Institutions for Handicapped Children* (London: Routledge and Kegan Paul).

Knights, D. & Morgan, G. (1990) 'The concept of strategy in sociology: a note of dissent', *Sociology* 24, 3, 475–83.

Lynaugh, J. (1988) 'Twice as many: and still not enough', *Secretary's Commission in Nursing. Support Studies and Background Information*. Vol. II. (Bethesda MD: Department of Health and Human Services).

Lynch, L. (1989) 'The nurses' strike at children's hospital drags on', *The East Bay Express*, 15 September, pp. 3, 8, 10.

McFarlane, J. K. (1976) 'A charter for caring', *Journal of Advanced Nursing*, 1, 187–96.

McFarlane, J. K. (1977) 'Developing a theory of nursing: the relation of theory to practice, education and research', in *Journal of Advanced Nursing*, 2, 261–70.

MacGuire, J. (1980) 'Nursing: none is held in higher esteem. Occupational control and the position of women in nursing', in Silverstone, J. & Ward, A. (eds) *Careers of Professional Women* (London: Croom Helm).

Macmillan, P. (1980) 'Major implications', *Nursing Times*, 76, 49, 2138–9.

Melia, K. M. (1982) '"Tell it as it is" – qualitative methodology and nursing research: understanding the student nurses' world', *Journal of Advanced Nursing*, 7, 327–35.

Melia, K. M. (1984) 'Student nurses' construction of occupational socialisation', *Sociology of Health and Illness*, 6, 2, 132–49.

Melia, K. M. (1987) *Learning and Working: The Occupational Socialization of Nurses* (London: Tavistock).

Menzies, I. E. P. (1960) 'A case study of the functioning of social systems as a defence against anxiety. A report on the study of a nursing service of a general hospital', *Human Relations*, 13, 95–121.

Miller, A. & Gwynn, G. (1972) *A Life Apart* (London: Tavistock).

Mohammed, S. (1986) 'A black perspective', *Senior Nurse*, 5, 3, 5.

Moores, B. & Moult, A. (1979) 'Patterns of nurse activity', *Journal of Advanced Nursing*, 4, 137–49.

Norton, D. (1962) *Investigation of geriatric nursing problems in hospitals* (Edinburgh: Churchill Livingstone).

O'Brien, M. (1989) 'Reproducing the world', in *Reproducing the World: Essays in Feminist Theory* (USA: Westview Press).

Oakley, A. (1981) 'Interviewing women: a contradiction in terms', in Roberts, H. (ed.) *Doing Feminist Research* (London: Routledge and Kegan Paul).

Oakley, A. (1984) 'The importance of being a nurse', *Nursing Times*, 80, 50, 24–7.

Ogier, M. (1982) *An Ideal Sister* (London: Royal College of Nursing).

Orton, H. D. (1981) *Learning Climate: A Study of the role of the Ward Sister in Relation to Student Nurse Learning on the Ward* (London: Royal College of Nursing).

Pearsall, M. (1970) 'Participant observation as role and method in behaviour', in Kilstead, W. J. (ed.) *Qualitative Methodology: Firsthand Involvement with the Social World* (Chicago: Markham).

Pearson, A. (ed.) (1988) *Primary Nursing: Nursing in the Burford and Oxford Nursing Development Units* (Beckenham: Croom Helm).

Pembrey, S. E. M. (1980) *The ward sister – key to nursing* (London: Royal College of Nursing).

Platzer, H. (1988) 'Redressing the balance', *Nursing Standard*, 2, 15, 42.

Price Waterhouse (1988) *Nurse Recruitment and Retention: Report on the factors affecting the Retention and Recruitment of Nurses, Midwives and Health Visitors in the NHS*. Commissioned by Chairmen of Regional Health Activities in England, Health Boards in Scotland and Health Authorities in Wales. (London: Price Waterhouse).

Proctor, S. (1989) 'The functioning of nursing routines in the management of a transient workforce', *Journal of Advanced Nursing*, 14, 180–9.

Revans, R. W. (1964) *Standards for Morale: Cause and Effect in Hospitals* (Oxford: Oxford University Press).

Roper, N. (1975) *Clinical Experience in Nurse Education: A Survey of the Available Nursing Experience for General Student Nurses in a School of Nursing in Scotland* (M.Phil. thesis: University of Edinburgh).

Roper, N. (1976) 'A model for nursing and nursology', *Journal of Advanced Nursing*, 1, 219–27.

Roper, N., Logan, W. & Tierney, A. (1985) 'The Roper/Logan/Tierney model', *Senior Nurse*, 3, 2, 20–6.

Salvage, J. (1985) *The Politics of Nursing* (London: Heinemann).

Salvage, J. (1990) 'The theory and practice of the "New Nursing"', *Nursing Times*, Occasional Paper, 86, 4, 42–5.

Salvage, J. and Kershaw, B. (eds) (1990) *Models for Nursing 2* (London: Scutari Press).

Shaw, M. (1990) 'Debate on the concept of strategy. Strategy and social process: military context and sociological analysis', *Sociology*, 24, 3, 465–73.

Sheehan, J. (1983) 'Educating for teaching nursing', in Davis, B. D. (ed.) *Research into Nurse Education* (London: Croom Helm).

Smith, P. (1987) 'The relationship between quality of nursing care and the ward as a learning environment: developing a methodology', *Journal of Advanced Nursing*, 12, 413–20.

Sontag, S. (1983) *Illness as Metaphor* (Harmondsworth: Penguin).

Stacey, M. (1981) 'The division of labour revisited or overcoming the two Adams', in Abrams, P., Deem, R., Finch, J. & Rock, P. (eds) *Practice and Progress: British Sociology 1950–1980* (London: Allen and Unwin).

Stanley, L. & Wise, S. (1983) *Breaking Out: Feminist Consciousness and Feminist Research* (London: Routledge and Kegan Paul).

Stockwell, F. (1972) *The Unpopular Patient* (London: Royal College of Nursing).

Strauss, A. L. & Glaser, B. G. (1970) *Anguish: A Case History of a Dying Trajectory* (London: Martin Robinson).

Strauss, A., Fagerhaugh, S., Suczek, B. & Wiener, C. (1982*a*) 'The work of hospitalised patients', *Social Science and Medicine*, 16, 977–86.

Strauss, A., Fagerhaugh, S., Suczek, B. & Wiener, C. (1982*b*) 'Sentimental work in the technologized hospital', *Sociology of Health and Illness*, 4, 3, 254–78.

Sullivan, V. (1989) 'Nursing's Rx: redefine the profession to the public', *UC Focus*, 3, 7, 3.

Tronto, J. C. (1987) 'Beyond gender difference to a theory of care', *Signs: Journal of Women in Culture and Society*, 12, 4, 644–63.

Ungerson, C. (1983*a*) 'Why do women care?', in Finch, J. & Groves, D. (eds) *A Labour of Love: Women, Work and Caring* (London: Routledge and Kegan Paul).

Ungerson, C. (1983*b*) 'Women and caring: skills, tasks and taboos', in Gamarnikov, E., Morgan, D., Purvis, J. & Taylorson, D. (eds) *The Public and the Private* (London: Heinemann).

Ungerson, C. (1990) 'The language of care', in Ungerson, C. (ed.) *Gender and Caring* (London: Harvester/Wheatsheaf).

United Kingdom Central Council for Nursing, Midwifery and Health Visiting Educational Policy Advisory Committee (1985) *Project 2000: Facing the Future. Project Paper 6* (London: UKCC).

United Kingdom Central Council for Nursing, Midwifery and Health Visiting (1986) *Project 2000: A New Preparation for Practice* (London: UKCC).

United Kingdom Central Council for Nursing, Midwifery and Health Visiting (1990) *The Post-Registration Education and Practice Project (PREPP)* (London: UKCC).

Webb, C. (1984*a*) 'On the eighth day God created the nursing process and nobody rested!', *Senior Nurse*, 1, 33, 22–5.

Webb, C. (1984*b*) 'Feminist methodology in nursing research', *Journal of Advanced Nursing*, 9, 249–50.

Index

oncology wards   55, 58
  compared with
    ophthalmology
    wards   56
overdose victims *see* drug
  abusers

participant
  observation   146–7,
  149, 153, 155
patient–nurse
  perceptions   40–2
patients
  dying   96–7, 98, 99, 100–3,
    105–7, 110
  elderly   86–7
  women   54, 60–1
  men   63
  nurses' attitudes to   41, 48,
    60–3, 71, 91, 112–13,
    144, 203–4
  effect of gender on   62–3
  role of   41
  violent   63–5, 67
  women   61–2
personal relationships   130
preceptors   143
primary nursing   9, 140
Project 2000   9, 19, 137–8,
  139, 141, 198
psychiatric wards   45–6, 56,
  200–1
  compared with other
    wards   57

questionnaire   20, 69, 54, 56,
  86, 90, 125, 149, 150,
  153–4, 156–7, 162–5
  findings   179–92
  see also survey; research

race   204
racial prejudice/
  stereotyping   66, 199
recruitment   81, 137
  advertisements   2–5, 11–13
research
  duration of   148–50
  organisation of   148–50
  exploratory   149
  see also data analysis; data
    collection; document
    analysis; interviews;
    questionnaire;
    survey
respiratory arrest   70
Ronda, Sister   87–9, 90, 92–3,
  124
  students' attitudes to   88,
    90

sentimental work   203
sexuality   63, 64, 67
sister   94, 204, 206–7
  allocation of work to
    students   75–6, 78,
    82
  caring   74, 75
  hierarchical   79
  ideal   27–8, 69
  management style   70–4,
    77, 78, 79, 80–1,
    88–9, 93, 133, 134,
    141; *see also* ward
    management style
  supportive   70–1, 73–4,
    128, 129
  traditional image   68–9
  unsupportive   72, 73–4, 79
sociology, feminist   147–8,
  198

219

specialties, medical 52, 59, 64
  legitimisation of emotion work by 55
  'pecking order' 53
statistical methods 157–9
stress 14, 58, 59, 71, 105, 126, 127
  see also anxiety
student nurses
  academic standards *see* educational qualifications
  changes in 112–13, 115, 125
  experience, variation in 100, 104, 119
  first-year 112–16, 120–1, 133
  'moulded' 27–9, 49–50, 129, 130
  selection of 22–6, 31–2
  supportive 128
  third-year 116–18, 124, 127
    taking examinations 118
    expectations of 119–20, 128
  typical 20–1, 25
  variations in expectation of 104
  within hierarchy *see* hierarchical relationships
  workforce, part of 33
support, emotional 43, 45, 140
surface acting 7, 15, 206
survey 57–8, 126–8
  see also questionnaire

talking to patients 89, 91, 106
time, male concept of 85, 89, 204
training 202
  content of 35–7, 52, 178
  course philosophy 175–7
  lack of 60, 132
  plan of 166–7
  relation to medical specialties 52, 53, 67
  theory vs practice 139

USA, nursing in 138

violent patients *see* patients, violent

ward allocation 202
ward handovers 92, 109
  examples 92–3, 106
ward management
  style 122–6, 133
  variations in 122, 127–8
ward placement, change of 119, 122–3, 125, 142
wards
  nurses' attitudes to 53, 54–5
  types of 52, 53
ward sister *see* sister
warehousing 193
Windermere, Sister 89, 126–7
women's work 18, 136, 195
  'natural' 2, 135